Fitz Koehler

YOUR HEALTHY CANCER COMEBACK

SICK *TO* STRONG

Fitzness Books

A division of Fitzness International LLC

Fitzness is a registered trademark of Fitz Koehler
and Fitzness International LLC
Gainesville, FL

Your Healthy Cancer Comeback: From Sick to Strong

For information or large orders, visit Fitzness.com
@Fitzness on Instagram, Facebook, and Youtube

Manufactured in the United States of America
Library of Congress Cataloging-in-Publication Data Available

Koehler, Fitz
Your Healthy Cancer Comeback: From Sick to Strong

Fitzness International LLC non-fiction original softcover
1. Health & Fitness / Diseases / Cancer
2. Health & Fitness / Healing
3. Health & Fitness / Exercise / General

Cover Designer: Melissa Redon
Layout Designer: Melissa Redon
Editor: Alicia Wilcox
Exercise photos were taken by: Phil Stokes
Photo Editor: Omar Benitez
Supplemental photos by: Omar Benitez and Jeremy Taylor

Contributing editors: Rudy Novotny

Proofreader: Doug Thurston and Jennifer Jeffres Sen

ISBN 978-1-7355998-5-4

YouR HeAltHy CaNCeR CoMebaCK

SICK *TO* STRONG

Fitz Koehler, MSESS

FITZNESS BOOKS

A DIVISION OF FITZNESS INTERNATIONAL LLC

I dedicate this book to
cancer crushers everywhere.
You can do hard things!

Contents

CHAPTER ONE

CONtRol

Instead of playing cancer's victim, you've chosen to do whatever it takes to fight for a healthy body, and this will be, by far, one of the most powerful decisions you'll ever make—not because of cancer, but despite cancer. Mental and physical strength, combined with knowledge and determination, will make you an unstoppable force. You know that physical weakness has no reward, and the more intelligent effort you put into your body, the more control over the outcomes you'll have. And that's why you picked up this book. You will not settle for sickness, weakness, and all of the other burdens cancer can bring. Come hell or high water, you will be healthy, strong, and fit. Your healthy cancer comeback awaits!

Cancer is infuriating. We've all been affected by it in one way or another. Whether you've had it yourself or your loved ones have gone through it, nobody is immune to experiencing its harsh effects. If you're reading this because you have been diagnosed with cancer, I'm gnashing my teeth for you. It's horrible, and I'm sorry you're stuck enduring the cure. However, the bright side is that most early-stage cancers are highly curable. Thanks to those who fund, conduct, and implement research, most cancer patients will eventually hear the word "remission." Breast cancer, for example, boasts more than a 90-percent cure rate. While this number is still not at all acceptable for a disease that targets one out of every eight women, that high survival rate is pretty encouraging. For those living with metastatic cancer, a commitment to your health can increase your quality of life and longevity. In fact, a study at Tel Aviv University, published in the November 2022 *Cancer Research* journal, found that high-intensity aerobic exercise can reduce the risk of metastatic cancer by 72-percent.[1] If this isn't a compelling argument to get moving, I don't know what is!

A cancer diagnosis can leave you feeling like your life is spinning out of control, and during this chaotic time, one of the main things we wish for is control. My transition from healthy and athletic to cancer patient with endless appointments and a "fall risk" bracelet on my arm was quick, confusing, and overwhelmingly stressful. But as I learned, I had—and you have—way more control than you think. And controlling the things that you can is going to enhance your calm, confidence, courage, and overall experience.

For example, you choose your doctors, and you choose whether or not to accept their treatment plans. Finding doctors you believe are intelligent, capable, and accomplished is going to give you far more confidence than being "assigned" a doctor, right? When you walk into oncology, it's important that you have faith in the person managing your survival. I was mesmerized by my oncologist's intellect during my bout with breast cancer, which yielded trust and faith that his treatment plan would cure me. It did. If you don't believe in the first doctor you meet, seek out recommendations and consult with others until you connect with one. Getting second and third opinions does not make you difficult, it makes you diligent. Good doctors should facilitate this for you.

You also have control over the treatments you do or do not accept. Remember that you do not have to blindly go along with all of your doctor's suggestions. Your power to say "yes" or "no" keeps you in charge of the process and will make you feel less like a victim. You are in control of yourself.:no one else.

Mind you, I accepted 100 percent of my doctors' recommendations because I trusted them and reviewed the research. Controlling my care was critical when it came to keeping my mental health in check. Even if you always say "yes," know that you are granting permission to proceed. Final decisions are always yours.

There are many other things we can control during treatment that are statistically proven to increase health, happiness, and overall survival rates while decreasing recurrence rates. Exercise, for example, has many powerful benefits for those battling cancer.

Health Benefits of Exercise:

- Boosts your immune system
- Maintains muscle mass
- Increases strength
- Prevents weakness
- Increases stamina
- Decreases fatigue/boosts energy
- Increases flexibility
- Decreases tightness/soreness
- Increases balance
- Prevents falls
- Boosts your mood
- Decreases brain fog

- Decreases anxiety and depression
- Boosts self-confidence
- Improves sleep
- Maintains coordination
- Helps maintain a healthy weight
- Benefits skin
- Improves bone density
- Prevents osteoporosis
- Supports digestion
- Strengthens your heart and lungs
- Offers an opportunity for socialization
- Enhances your sexual confidence and enjoyment
- Keeps you engaged with your communities
- Increases survival rates for many cancers
- Decreases odds of recurrence

The concept of exercising during cancer care may seem outrageous, but I assure you that it's not as difficult as you might think. Millions of cancer patients stay active throughout their treatment to varying degrees, and there is an enormous amount of research proving its benefits. I have no crystal ball to know precisely what each one of my readers is going through, but I can assure you that if you commit to putting your best foot forward with exercise, nutrition, quality sleep, and stress management, along with perspective, passions, and positivity, your life will be enhanced during and after treatments. Everyone's path is different, and I don't expect you to run 10 miles each day (unless you want to), but incorporating some type of exercise into your routine has undeniable benefits. Within these pages, I will guide you toward doing better and being better. Progress will look different to each of you. Just fight this fire with fire and control as many of your outcomes and daily experiences as possible.

Cancer treatment is no joke. Obviously. But unless you've gone through it or are going through it, there's almost no way to thoroughly comprehend what the treatment triathlon —chemo, radiation, and surgeries— can do to a person. And that's on top of a ridiculous number of other innovative scans, tests, and treatments, as well as costs of care, which are often much greater than expected. It's a lot, and that's the understatement of the century.

Even if you're "only" enduring one form of treatment and escaping the others … the hardships can be mind-boggling. Physically and mentally, the cure for this disease is often brutal. It's worth it, of course, because the great majority of patients become survivors, but you are wise to pursue an intelligent strategy for a return to normalcy.

According to a report by the U.S. Department of Health and Human Services, exercise is associated with a 40- to 50-percent reduced disease-specific and overall mortality rate among patients diagnosed with breast, colorectal, or prostate cancer.[2] Pretty impressive, huh? Exercise can literally save your life. And isn't it empowering to be able to increase your survival chances with measures that have zero nasty, punishing, or painful side effects? I think so.

My attitude during treatment was to do every little positive thing I could so I wouldn't ever look back with regret. Would I take a pill called Tamoxifen for 10 years for a 1.2 percent extra likelihood I'd be around to see my kids get married? You betcha. But I was warned that Tamoxifen might come with negative side effects. On the flip side, there are no negative side effects to walking, dancing, or swimming daily for 30 minutes. Not that I'm aware of!

That's why we're here. The opportunity to take control of your health, your body, and your life is pretty splendid. I'm excited to help you expertly design your strategy for a body that works, a body you feel great in, and a body you love!

I still can't believe I had breast cancer. I also can't believe that I endured the dreaded cures for it. Chemo, radiation, surgeries … all of it. I'm a fitness expert and professional race announcer, and I make my living being a beacon of health. It's very strange to wrap my head around the fact that I was ever so sick, weak, bald, scared, and hurt. I bet you struggle with that too. But the reality is that I went through it, and I got through it. You can too, and I can help. It's funny, upon my diagnosis, I was given an hour-long Breast Cancer 101 lecture by my oncologist's nurse practitioner. Great gal, I really liked her. But looking back inspires a few thoughts.

1. She gave me a long list of possibilities of awful things that might happen during treatment, but most of the things she shared with me never happened.

2. A ton of strange side effects she never mentioned did occur, all of which shocked the heck out of me.

3. We never discussed the benefits of exercise during treatment.

4. We never discussed the benefits of nutrition during treatment.

5. We discussed treatment plans but didn't discuss the massive benefits of committing to fitness during care. They might have skipped this stuff because they knew what I did professionally, but it's a conversation that I think should be had in all circumstances. After all, this one conversation has the power to save your life, which is why you and I are having it right now.

Here's the deal. With cancer or without cancer, your health habits always matter. Let me repeat that: Your health habits always matter! The things you put into your body will always have an effect. They will affect you as you consume them, and they will have some sort of long-term effect. Whether they have a good effect or a bad effect depends on the foods and beverages you choose. The way you move your body will also have consequences. You can choose an active lifestyle filled with deliberate exercise, leading to strength, mobility, great balance, and stamina. Or, you can choose a sedentary lifestyle that will cause you to be weak, tight, unsteady, and breathless. I'm guessing you'll find the first option the most appealing. It is to me.

For the great majority of those I guide toward living better and longer with fitness or Fitzness (my particular brand of fitness), I teach a #noexcuses mentality. "Figure it out! Make plans and keep them!" I leave little room for failure as these strategies are fool-proof! When it comes to being a cancer patient, though, many of us legitimately lose lots of options. So, I lighten up a little bit. Yep, some of us have or had legitimate excuses not to exercise. For many of us, our food options become limited too. Perhaps a volatile tummy or deadened taste buds play the nemesis. Surgery could be an obstacle. Fair enough. So, what I'm going to provide here is guidance from which you can choose the options that work for you. I know that health goals, especially during cancer treatment, are never one-size-fits-all, which is why I'm here to guide you on your individual path and give you advice that you can implement in your own way. Your goal should be to maintain whatever fitness level you have and work to improve it as you can. Wisely. Gently. Consistently.

Much like snowflakes and fingerprints, every cancer case is unique. Even within particular types of cancer (brain, ovarian, colon, etc), very few cancer patients walk an identical path. I can and have been in rooms with 100 other breast cancer survivors and not one of us shared a uniform experience. Did you know that there are many different "types" of breast cancer? The same goes for brain cancer, blood cancer, and others. Think about it. Cancers vary by genetic makeup, tumor sizes, tumor locations, tumor quantities … and more. I remind you of this so that you do not compare yourself to others. You just can't. Instead, I want you to set very specific goals for yourself. Your friend's dad's cousin who had the same kind of cancer as you? Not relevant.

Within these pages, we'll discuss both your physical and mental fitness and how to make the best of each. Keep in mind that not only am I not a doctor, but even if I was, I would not be YOUR doctor. So, take this information specifically as guidance from a fitness expert to help you choose a path back toward fitness. You and your doctor should be making 100-percent of the official calls on your medical decisions. Nothing in this book should be considered medical advice. Instead, remember that I am a highly qualified, high-caliber fitness pro who's got major street-cred as a cancer survivor. I was obliterated by treatment and then strategically orchestrated my return to impressive strength, stamina, athleticism, and happiness. I meticulously designed my workouts at the start of my treatment, pulled back for rest and recovery during many months during my "mean chemo," and gently yet aggressively pursued improvements in fitness as my body allowed. I want the same for you. In fact, I wrote this book because while I was working my way back from sick to strong, I couldn't stop thinking about how fortunate I was to be a fitness expert. I was so weak and so scrawny, just a shadow of my former self. I knew that if I didn't have this lifetime of education and experience in my head, my recovery might have seemed impossible. My heart broke for my peers fighting similar battles without all of the know-how. Helping you go from sick to strong may be one of the most important and valuable things I ever do professionally. I'm so excited to help.

Let's get you back to your pre-cancer health status … and then take you further. After all, the second you heard those horrific words, "you have cancer," the only thing you wished for was your health. Whether you prioritized it before or not, now you do. Your healthy cancer comeback awaits!

CHAPTER TWO

MeNtal FiTNeSS wiTH tHe tHRee P's

Before we focus on your body, let's get your head on straight.

Your most enthusiastic coach and cheerleader is going to have to be the voice in your head, because controlling how you view and respond to cancer care will be essential to your success. I talked a bunch about the "three P's" (Perspective, Passions, and Positivity) in my memoir *My Noisy Cancer Comeback: Running at the Mouth While Running for My Life* and these are the things readers constantly tell me they're still using today, even after their healthy cancer comeback has arrived! They also thank me for sharing so many absurd stories that made them laugh at me and allowed them to laugh at themselves. Note: This cancer nonsense can often be funny.

Perspective

Many years ago I was standing in the "10 items or less" checkout lane at my local grocery store and in a hurry. Unfortunately for me, the 353-year-old woman ahead of me was removing about 4,052 items from her cart and paying for them with a check. So frustrating! Of course, I would never say anything disrespectful or give cranky vibes to a senior, but on the inside,

I was stewing. That is until I looked over to aisle #2. Standing there was a teeny little 5-year-old-ish girl wearing a shiny red, blue, and yellow Snow White dress and a very bald head. It pained me to imagine what that poor child must be going through. And then I thought about how much her parents must be suffering.

Instantly, I was so grateful that my greatest burden in life was having to wait patiently in line at the grocery store. I was suddenly embarrassed for feeling so irritated by it. And that perspective has stuck with me ever since. In fact, "it's not cancer" became my mantra. If I lost an expensive piece of technology, I'd think "it's not cancer!", and I'd be over it in an instant. If someone canceled on me or I lost a work opportunity, "it's not cancer" and I'd move on. When most people stuck in a massive traffic jam are grousing angrily, I'm the weirdo who can only focus on how grateful I am not to be the person in the accident that caused the jam. This perspective has saved me endless amounts of self-induced misery over the years and I'm grateful for it.

On February 26, 2019, when my doctor called me to tell me I had cancer, I struggled. I cried, I feared and I certainly thought I was a goner. My stress was agonizing. But once I met with my oncologist who gave me guidance and hope, I decided to take control of the things that I could. The first thing on my agenda was to reenlist my mighty sidekick: PERSPECTIVE. Sure, I actually was dealing with cancer this time - ouch! But the bright side for me was that I wasn't a kid with cancer, and better yet, it wasn't MY kid with cancer. Short of that, I decided to don my big-girl panties and soldier on. Did I cry? Every single day. Usually alone in my bathroom or car. But I'd boo-hoo as much as I needed to, and then wipe my tears, put on the best smile I could, and go conquer my day.

Perspective will prevent the stress of cancer from eating you alive. Your brain is a powerful weapon in this fight and you must steer it in the direction of strength and hope. Allow your grief to come out, but don't allow yourself to live in a state of grief. There will always be something to be grateful for, and there will always be something to smile about. Sometimes you just have to look for it.

Passions

I was blown away by how impactful my choice to pursue my passions during treatment became. I couldn't control the fact that I had cancer, but I could control the way that I responded to it. So one of the first things I decided for myself was that no matter what, cancer was not going to keep me from the career that I built and adored, nor special times with my kids. Ginger and Parker were 15 and 13 respectively, and I decided that regardless of what was happening with my health, if they had a game, performance, graduation, or any other special event, I was going to be there. I also decided that I wasn't going to miss the races I announced or keynote speaking opportunities. My race announcing calendar alone had me flying around the country (about 30 trips) to host massive running events like the Los Angeles Marathon, Buffalo Marathon, and Big Sur Marathon. Does that sound crazy for a cancer patient? Maybe. But to me, it was my lifeblood. After all, I earned my rightful spot on those stages and I did not want to give up my position or my income. I loved my work and knew that if I stayed home missing all of the events and people I adored, I would just cry all weekend. Clearly, that wouldn't be beneficial to my health at all.

When I made these decisions, I had no idea what I was in for. I never imagined I'd become so violently ill that I'd require IV fluids every single weekday for five months. I didn't know I'd end up sleeping on hotel bathroom floors regularly because my rooms felt like they wouldn't stop spinning. But I also couldn't have fathomed what magic awaited. I'd come to know that when I picked myself off of those floors, got dressed, and got on stage, almost all of those nasty side effects would disappear. I had no way of knowing that the greatest cure for the horribleness I was experiencing was to be with the people that I love doing the things that I love. It was phenomenal. No matter what hardship or trauma my body was going through, when I stepped up to the microphone, I got to be full-force Fitz Koehler again. The adrenaline and joy superseded my sickness and pain allowing me to have huge chunks of time where I felt magnificent. The same goes for special times with my kids. Watching and celebrating their accomplishments removed me from my own situation and encouraged me to enjoy theirs. Glorious.

Your passions are important and I implore you to commit to them right now! Whatever they are, you must find a way to incorporate them into your life in any and every way possible. They will fuel you, distract you, and keep a certain amount of joy in your life that will prove to be invaluable over time.

Do you love soccer? Great! Go kick a ball. If you're feeling too tired to play, go watch other people play. If you're stuck in the hospital or at home in bed, watch soccer on television, read about the latest matches, or get on the phone and discuss it with your best mate. You can always immerse yourself in your favorite sport if you're committed.

Perhaps you are crazy about animals? Me too! You'll find your pets to be an incredible source of comfort and happiness at this time. They don't know what's going on, they just want your attention and affection. My lab-mix Piper rarely left my side when I was sick at home. She loved the amount of sitting, sleeping, and cuddling I was doing. It's actually been proven, time and time again, that mere physical touch with your pets increases the level of serotonin in your brain. If you don't have your own pets, ask friends to stop by with theirs or visit a local farm, zoo, or animal shelter. Stuck in a chair all day for chemo? Watch funny animal videos on the internet or ask for a service animal to come to visit your room. There are so many options.

Hopefully, you have a couple of things that instantly popped into your head when I mentioned your passions. If so, add them to the calendar on your phone as a daily reminder. You don't have to book times right now, just put those words in as a recurring "appointment" each day so you'll constantly be prompted to take action. If you're not instinctively coming up with ideas, that's fine. Just make a simple list of things you enjoy. Books, knitting, cars, cooking, music, crafts, puzzles, etc. Build your passions into your world consistently. I promise they will have a major impact on your overall well-being.

Positivity

I discovered early on that I got zero extra points for being the saddest girl in the room. Being miserable had no benefit. Is it justified to feel sad, stressed, and scared? Abso-freaking-lutely! Is it beneficial to laser focus on those feelings and carry them around like a badge of honor? Heck no! Folks, if cancer does anything really well, it helps us focus on the important things in life: health and happiness. Health is what you're fighting for. Happiness, though, you can have it right now. Right now! Cancer can take away a lot of things, but it shouldn't take away your ability to enjoy your loved ones, music, jokes, a beautiful day, puppy kisses, and more.

Do you have friends on social media or in real life who are always sharing negatives? I see this post constantly. "Pray for me. I sprained my ankle." And then the following comments are of pity and commiseration ... all over a merely twisted ankle. I'm curious why anyone would want to eat up all the prayers on a sprained ankle, and also why anyone would beg for this type of attention. If I fell and sprained my ankle I would not want to broadcast the fall, unless it came from hilarious circumstances. "An alligator ran out from under my Jeep as I was climbing out and I sprained my ankle trying not to step directly into his open mouth!" That's a story worth sharing. But really - our friends who show up with endless complaints aren't adding positive energy to their lives or yours.

With cancer, you'll likely have lots of difficult moments to harp on, and sharing them with a close confidant and/or a counselor can be helpful. But I assure you, if you focus on how helpful those nasty chemo drugs are going to be - you might be a little less angry at them. If you consider how sweet the nurse who stuck you with that needle was, you might feel happy and hopeful because your medical team sincerely cares. If you share a few fun or funny photos of you and your newly bald head, you might hear from friends who think you look fabulous! Instead of dwelling on your suffering, try to find the good, happiness, and fun in every situation. Am I Susie Sunshine about life? Possibly. But it is much easier and far more delightful to focus on the positive whenever possible. I encourage you to seek out the hilarity in many of your preposterous situations. Patients who can laugh at themselves are simply having a happier time despite their diagnosis. Yes, you have cancer. But yes you can still laugh, play and enjoy!

Besides committing to Perspective, Passions, and Positivity, I have one more weapon in this mental war that will help you endure the hard stuff and conquer your challenges more effectively. I stumbled across this useful tool right before my treatment began. One of my last obligations before starting chemo was to get an MRI. For most folks, it's simply a measure of lying still inside a machine while it takes pictures of your innards. Some have referred to the experience as "relaxing." I hope this is your experience. But if you're claustrophobic like me, lying face down on the little bed and being shoved into the machine while Thor bangs his hammer on the outside of it comes with some extreme challenges. In fact, for me, it became chaotic. After a full-blown freakout during which I screamed and flailed and demanded escape from the machine, the MRI lady reset me and gave me one more chance to try it again. This came under the stern warning that if we weren't successful in getting images today, I could not start chemo and the cancer-killing would not begin. As she slid me back into the machine for 45 minutes, I started talking to myself and that internal conversation became a nonstop pep-talk. I kept running through all of the difficult challenges I'd conquered in my life. I've raised two wonderful children. I've built an international business. I competed in full-contact kickboxing for almost 10 years. "I can do hard things!" Those five words I said to myself over and over and over. Is that a bit crazy? Possibly. But did it work? Perfectly. I was able to talk myself into overcoming my fear, and I remained face-down in that tiny space until the task was complete.

That MRI machine was the place where I learned that if I wanted to survive, I was going to have to do a lot of things that scared me. And so each time I sat down for a needle poke, a scan, chemotherapy, radiation, or surgery I reminded myself that "I can do hard things." I must have repeated this a thousand times. Eventually, I had said it enough that all the scary procedures were over and I was cancer-free. Now, everything in life feels comparatively easy and when I'm faced with challenges in business or my personal life, these things seem trivial.

Perspective
Passions
Positivity

"I Can Do Hard Things!"

CHAPTER THREE

FOUR PILLARS OF FITNESS

Before we delve into pursuing fitness during cancer care, let's quickly go over the vital components of fitness.
Once you understand how undeniably-essential each pillar is and how to pursue each, your confidence and outcomes with exercise will skyrocket. Even if you have spent your entire life as a fitness superstar, humor me please, and read on. I often say that I have a master's degree in the most simple stupid science on the planet (Exercise and Sport Sciences), but you'd be amazed by how many people find it confusing or miss out on vital elements. Fitness may seem as simple as "go for a walk", but it's not. On the flip side, it's also not as complicated as having to count carbs and compete in triathlons. Right now we're going to stick purely to the exercise components of fitness.

Four Pillars of Fitness

To qualify as physically fit, you've got to put in some effort and see results in four different categories: strength, cardio-respiratory endurance, flexibility, and balance. I call them the Four Pillars of Fitness because each is a vital component of physical fitness and without even one element, the roof could cave in. Yes, even if you're an athlete. Ask yourself if the following people are truly fit:

1. A marathon runner who doesn't have the strength to do five push-ups or carry his luggage.

2. A body-building champion, who can't touch her toes or reach behind her to scratch her own back.

3. A yoga instructor who becomes breathless after climbing two flights of stairs.

4. A competitive swimmer who can't stand on one foot for 30 seconds without falling.

The answer to all four examples is NO. None of them meet the criteria to qualify as fit. This is important to understand because too many people laser-focus on one or maybe two areas of fitness and completely neglect the others.

As a cancer patient, maintaining each pillar will benefit you significantly. Treatment may leave you weaker, stiffer, fatigued, and wobbly. If you work toward strength, stamina, mobility, and balance , you may be able to counteract some of the nasty effects while preventing extra problems such as falls, sprains, strains, tears, or bone breaks. I strongly recommend saving yourself from extra misery wherever and whenever you can.

And here's some fantastic news: not every cancer patient ends up sick, frail, and listless. I have friends who are doing extraordinary things while going through various types of cancer treatments. My girls Vikki and Angela are running 30-plus miles per week while enduring the same chemo treatments that rendered me violently ill. Everyone responds differently to their care, and you may be one of the superstars who actually thrives in this tricky time. Why not? Your cancer diagnosis may be just the motivation you needed to get fit and stay fit forever. I support that. Going back to those Four Pillars of Fitness, let's do a deeper dive so you completely understand each and are prepared to pursue them.

Muscular Strength

This is your body's ability to lift, push, pull, press, and move in other ways. Muscular strength can be improved with all sorts of exercises in which you move your body against resistance. Body weight exercises such as squats, lunges, pushups, calf raises, crunches, and bridges are great choices because they require zero equipment and utilize gravity to make you stronger. Using tools such as free weights, bands, cables, kettlebells, plyo-boxes, and medicine balls will add variety and challenges to your training.

Cardio-Respiratory Endurance

This references the power of your heart and lungs to efficiently pump blood throughout your body and process oxygen. The stronger these organs are, the easier breathing will be at rest and at work. You can enhance cardio-respiratory endurance via exercises that make you huff and puff. Running, cycling, swimming, dancing, jumping, kicking, and boxing are some great examples. Aerobic activity is done at a pace at which you huff and puff but can keep exercising for an extended period. Running at a moderate pace, for example, is preferable to sprinting a short distance and stopping.

Flexibility

This is your body's ability to bend, reach and twist through a wide range of motions. You should target all muscles in your body for this benefit. Increased flexibility will allow you to extend your body parts in various directions without risking sprains, strains, and tears. It will also help you avoid the aches and pains that stem from stiffness. Cancer care often requires lots of rest which leads to muscle stiffness and soreness. Prioritize stretching multiple times each day and pursue workouts like yoga and tai chi. If movement becomes extremely difficult, you can even stretch in bed and in the shower. Even tiny bits here and there can make a positive impact.

Balance Training

Do this and you'll be less likely to fall down. That's a simple explanation, right? Sure, you've probably gone your whole adult life without face-planting like a drunken sailor. I got it. But this new phase is likely going to be different. Chemotherapy and other drugs can affect your brain, vision, and equilibrium, and can cause dehydration that makes you unsteady on your feet. Surgeries and amputations may steal your strength or complicate your ability to walk properly. Radiation and mobility limitations might affect your balance as well. Putting time into this pillar of fitness will enhance something called proprioception. That's basically your body's natural ability to respond to an imbalance without purposely thinking about it. If, for example, you step off of the sidewalk and onto the squishy grass while walking … with quality proprioception – your brain will instantly tell your ankle not to roll, it will hold its position and you won't fall. But without that practiced skill, you may go boom. Balance training can be done anywhere at any time.

Hopefully, you're convinced that each pillar of fitness is essential, and you are pledging to make progress in each. Without any of the four, you may find yourself paying a consequence you wish you hadn't.

The F.I.T.T. Principle

Frequency – how often should you exercise?

For a healthy individual, I'd suggest exercising most days of the week. For a cancer patient, I'd still suggest exercising most days of the week IF YOU

CAN! If you're bedridden and feeling horrible, do not. Remember, this is YOUR CALL. But I stand by my recommendation. If you can do something, do something! Deliberately exercising four to seven days a week is the gold standard. For those days when you just can't intentionally exercise, being active will go a long way. For those days that you can't be active, get the best rest possible. For those days when you need to rest, gently stretch in bed or the shower if you can. Every ounce of effort counts.

Intensity – how hard should you exercise?

Let's break this down pillar by pillar. Focus on the keywords: grunt, huff and puff, wince and wobble.

Strength: To become stronger, you should be lifting slightly more weight and/or doing more repetitions than you did previously. You should challenge your muscles to a point where they feel like they can no longer lift, press, push or pull. A good sign that you're working at an appropriate level is when you're induced to "grunt." If you choose to increase resistance, you will fatigue with fewer repetitions. If you do not increase resistance, you may not fatigue until you do significantly more reps.

Cardio: Increase your heart and lung capacity by doing exercises that make you huff and puff for extended periods. If you can walk and talk forever, you're likely not working hard enough to advance your cardio-respiratory capacity. If you are sprinting and can't squeak out "gee, this is so hard" you're working too hard. If you are moving your body at a maintainable pace that keeps you huffing and puffing, you're right in the zone.

Flexibility: Stretching performed after a vigorous workout is the best time to make progress and increase flexibility. This is because your core temperature has increased and your muscles are pliable. With any stretch, reach to the point that makes you "wince." You know the feeling where you think "Wooooh! I feel that!" Get to that point and hold your position for 10-20 seconds. Relax and repeat that stretch to see if you can go a little further. Reminder: Feeling the stretch is different from feeling pain. DO NOT push to pain or past it.

Stretching can also be beneficial in tiny increments throughout your day. You really can't overdo it, so bend, reach and twist as frequently as you can.

Balance: Balance can only be improved when you test it with something that makes you wobble. That's right: you improve your balance by doing things that put you off balance. Start in a place where you can easily hold on to something strong and stationary for support if necessary. Stand on one foot. If you wobble, work to hold that position for 30 seconds or for as long as you can. If you stand on one foot and do not wobble, try a more challenging move. Stand on one foot while flapping your arms. Stand on one foot while closing your eyes. When you feel your hips, knees, ankles, and feet shift a bit, you'll know that you're doing an appropriate exercise to make progress. Balance training is important. Falling down is no fun.

Whenever training for progress, remember to work at intensities that make you Huff-Puff, Grunt, Wince, and Wobble! If you're not aiming for progress and are simply hoping to maintain the capabilities you already have, just keep working at the same intensity and doing the things you can already do. Remember, you are in charge of yourself, so gauge your body daily and make decisions that are appropriate for the situation you're in.

Time – how long should you exercise?

For average folks, I suggest 30-minute to 90-minute sessions. This time range offers the opportunity to get your heart rate up and work on various body parts in various ways. In most circumstances, the more you do, the more significant your progress will be. But it's also true that short bits of exercise can be beneficial in a big way. Doing five minutes of jumping rope, lunges, or stretching will certainly be meaningful. All exercise counts, so never get hung up on the things you can't do or don't have time for. Instead, commit to doing what you can when you can, and results will follow.

Exercise newbies should start small and progress gradually. Choose a low-intensity workout and do it until you're satisfied. It's okay if you only exercise for five minutes in the beginning. You are where you are. When you return for the next workout session, do a little bit more than you did the first time. If you commit to gradual progress, you won't likely suffer the consequences of doing too much too soon which can be incredibly painful and defeating. Moderation is the secret to avoiding unnecessary setbacks which require time off for healing. Also, everyone's cancer comeback journey is different, so only base your progress on how much you're improving, not how well you're doing compared to anyone else.

Type - what kind of exercise?

Besides incorporating the Four Pillars of Fitness, it's a wise idea to vary your choices for exercise within each pillar. When you change up the type of exercise you do, your body has to adjust to the new challenge and will grow more capable because of it. If you only walk, for example, don't expect to be great at swimming or cycling. Think about the different ways your body moves with each of these three exercises and which muscles are utilized. There is a tremendous difference! If you mix up your routines, your body will benefit from the struggle to succeed.

I'll share a few different types of workouts within each Pillar of Fitness.

Cardio	Balance
Running	Standing on a pillow
Dancing	Tai Chi
Boxing	BOSU Exercises

Strength	Flexibility
Dumbbells	Yoga
Cable Machines	Martial Arts
Resistance Bands	Stretching with Bands

Overall, your routine mustn't become too "routine." Without expecting you to become a fitness wizard, continuously aim to try one new exercise or utilize a new piece of equipment each time you work out. The worst piece of equipment is the one you're not using, so make it your mission to give them all a go! Besides this book, you will find an infinite amount of free resources such as instructional workout videos, innovative training product recommendations, advice columns, and more on my website Fitzness.com.

Deliberate Exercise vs. Being Active

Besides committing to deliberate exercise, I also recommend you commit to an active lifestyle. What's the difference? Deliberate exercise is when you purposely set out to improve on at least one pillar of fitness. This often requires some sort of equipment: a sports bra, running shoes, tights, goggles, etc. It also usually causes a person to huff, puff, grunt, wince, or wobble. "Being active" simply infers being in motion. Cleaning, gardening, grocery shopping, and changing a car tire all fall into the category of "being active." I love this category! It's basically the alternative to being a couch potato. Staying active is not only beneficial physically, but it will also keep your mind stimulated and prevent you from sitting around pondering all of the what-ifs. Rest is incredibly important and we're going to discuss that too. But for right now, commit to being active whenever possible and exercising in a way that makes you better.

Are You Brand New to Exercise?

If you've completely avoided deliberate exercise for a very long time, that's okay! There is no reason you can't start right now. Even if you're overweight. Even if you're older. Even if you're feeling helpless, weak, sad, confused, cranky, etc, all you need to do is start with the commitment to control what you can and use this book to start making small bits of progress. Chapter 7 is packed with all sorts of instructional exercise photos and suggestions for things to try. Choose just one thing and give it a go for just one minute. When you're ready for more, choose one more thing and do that for one minute. Add more as you feel comfortable, and soon you'll be experiencing the benefits of a fitter body that feels better and can do more of the things you'd like it to!

CHAPTER FOUR

TRAINING DURING TREATMENT

It is well-documented that exercise benefits cancer patients in a variety of meaningful ways. I think it's imperative to understand why you should do what you can when you can.

Maintain or increase physical strength. Being strong will allow you to lift, carry, push or pull basic items like groceries, babies, or laundry without struggle. Strength will also help you lift yourself. Weakness often leads to injuries.

Mobility. Unflexible muscles are more likely to hurt and experience sprains, strains, and tears.

Balance. Without it, you're likely to fall.

Endurance. Many treatments lead to fatigue. Increased stamina benefits you at work, play, and everything in between.

Improved sleep. Cancer care can be exhausting. Exercise will help you sleep better and longer.

Decreased symptoms of depression. The feel-good endorphins created by exercise combat the feel-sad juju associated with cancer.

Reduced anxiety. Expelling the pent-up emotions inside you through exercise is an effective way to remove toxic feelings.

Improved mood. When you decrease stress and anxiety and increase the feelings of accomplishment, the world seems a lot rosier.

Decreased pain. Fitter bodies are less likely to be injured and more likely to avoid the pain associated with simple tasks like sitting or standing too long, sleeping in various positions, or suffering from asymmetries.

Higher Self-Esteem. The more positive things you do for yourself, the better you're going to feel about yourself. Simple measures such as a morning stretch, a walk around the park, or a few balance training exercises will inspire feelings of accomplishment and success.

Lowers the risk of cancer recurring. Fitter bodies are associated with stronger immune systems and are often far more capable of fighting off all sorts of illnesses, ailments, and diseases. Given the choice, an oncologist would likely favor the odds of a healthy and fit patient over an unfit one. Do not underestimate the power you have to preserve your own health.

Accountability Counts!

Avoid Too Much Rest

While loved ones may encourage you to rest constantly and avoid anything physically demanding, that advice may do more harm than good. Besides missing out on that big list of wonderful benefits fitness can provide, Dr. Dawn Mussallem, Breast Cancer Lifestyle Medicine Specialist, cautions that excessive sedentary time increases cancer risk, even for individuals who are putting in time exercising before or after work. She adds that a person who sits at a desk all day should set an alarm to get up and move a few minutes every 30 minutes.[3] This is the definition of squeezing in a little bit of activity. So simple!

Schedule It In

Just like everybody else, you should make specific plans to exercise. Whether you choose to do so before work, during the afternoon, or in the evenings, put it on your agenda each day and stick to it. Sign up for classes, make plans with friends, or choose a time and make it a habit. Obviously, there are going to be times where you unexpectedly feel too sick or tired to workout, and that's understandable. In that case, you don't have to schedule a particular workout in, you can just write down a list of exercises that you plan to accomplish that day or week. Then, when you're feeling up to it, you can tackle that to-do list. However, if you don't commit to moving your body ahead of time and hold yourself accountable, it's less likely to happen. Consider it "me time," the time when you take control over your health and decide what's going to happen with it. Increased strength, endurance, balance, and flexibility are on your calendar! This is the time when you fend off physical deterioration from treatment. Imagine how cool it's going to be when you put cancer behind you and can tell folks how you continued to exercise through it. You'll impress them, and impress yourself!

Working While Waiting

You're likely going to be stuck in a ton of waiting rooms and exam rooms during this time. The amount of sitting and waiting is almost comical. Throw in a few scans where you're required to be perfectly still and you're going to be MORE than eager to execute the following philosophies. As you wait, keep these simple principles in mind:

Standing is better than sitting.

Swaying or stepping side to side is better than standing still.

Moving vigorously is usually better than moving slowly.

Instead of just wasting time on your phone or "gasp!" Googling the horrible possibilities that may accompany your diagnosis – move! Be creative about it. You can do mundane movements in public places like standing, swaying, or walking, but when you get behind closed doors – let 'er rip! Dance, jump, squat, and do pushups on the wall or countertops. Just do SOMETHING. You can also take selfies posing glamorously in your fancy hospital gowns, make glove monsters, and draw pictures for your medical team on the paper covering the exam table. I did these things routinely. It ate up time, made me and my doctors giggle, and prevented me from getting stiff from sitting in chairs. If you do take any good "working while waiting" selfies – share them with me. PLEASE! I'm @Fitzness everywhere.

Exam Room Exercises

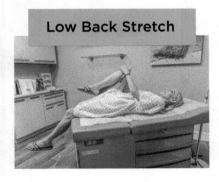

Low Back Stretch

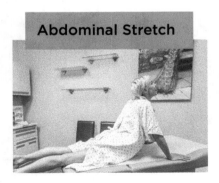

Abdominal Stretch

Squats

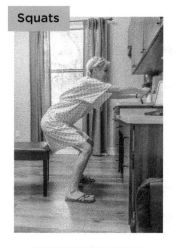

Push Ups

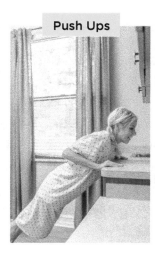

Calf Stretches

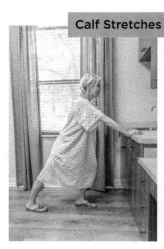

Back Stretches

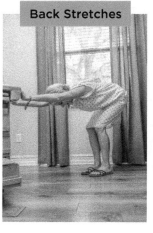

Side Planks

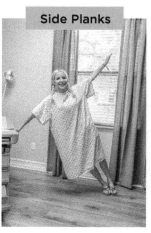

Hamstring Stretches

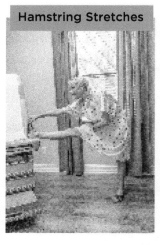

Hamstring Stretches

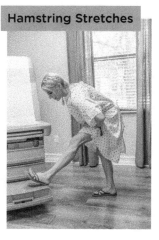

Hip Flexor Stretches

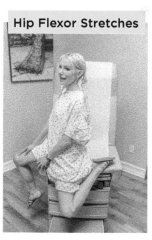

Dips

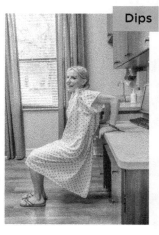

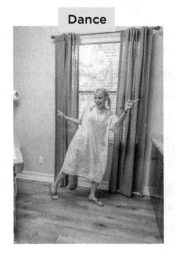

Dance

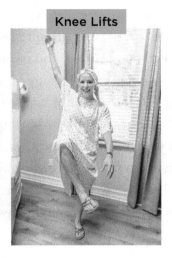

Knee Lifts

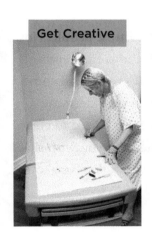

Get Creative

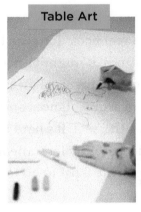

Table Art

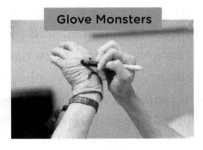

Glove Monsters

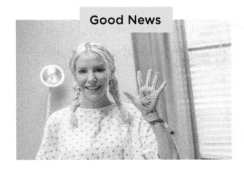

Good News

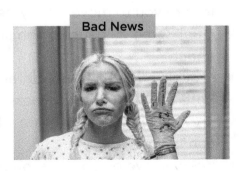

Bad News

Not all patients become terribly weak and/or sick. In fact, many feel well enough to run long distances, participate in adventurous sports and build muscle! It's been exciting to see many of my friends thriving while surviving. Perhaps you will end treatment fitter than you were when it began? Some people might suggest that's insanity. I think the concept is inspiring – and I've seen it happen with my own eyes. As you know, the second you heard the words "you have cancer," not much mattered other than your health. In that vein, it would be insane not to pursue improvements to the parts of your health that you can control. Your new or heightened respect for your body, health, and life may be just the thing that sets you on course to become the best you yet. I hope so.

Training Partners

Exercising with a buddy can be a real boost for even the fittest people. Now that you're going through hard times, it might be a wise idea to exercise with a buddy, trainer, or as part of an organized group. If you've had some friends, neighbors, and/or random acquaintances offer to provide some support – this might be a fun way to use it. It's hard to ask a friend to clean your toilets, although you should certainly let someone help you with that. But it's far less uncomfortable to invite a pal to go for walks, do a workout video together, or attend a yoga class.

Training partners can:

- Inspire you to move simply because they showed up.
- Offer some guidance on an activity they're knowledgeable about.
- Provide emotional support and encouragement.
- Entertain with great conversation and companionship.
- Try new workouts with you when you're not feeling confident.
- Keep an eye on you! Yes, on occasion you may need it.

Ouch Has No Place in Exercise

A simple rule of thumb that most physical therapists will agree on is that if an exercise causes pain, you should not do it. This will prevent you from harming yourself. You need to know the difference between pain and being challenged. Pain = "Ouch!" Productive exercise = "Gee this is hard!" If a movement causes pain, just choose a different movement that feels good. Make note of the painful motion and discuss it with your physician or physical therapist at your next appointment.

You also need to pull the plug on any exercise that makes you feel sick or dizzy. Those feelings come when your body has had enough. If you're on the brink of dizziness, find something stable to hold on to or sit down in a safe place while taking deep breaths to help you cool down gradually. Going from a fast pace to stationary is never a great idea, but falling down is a more critical risk than missing a smart cool-down.

If you feel nauseous, immediately slow down and take deep breaths. Hopefully, that feeling will subside without actual sickness occurring. And here's the deal. If you think that it's cool when elite athletes puke while training …maybe you're right. But exercise-induced nausea or vomiting during cancer treatment is not cool at all. It's dangerous. To keep you out of the danger zone while exercising, I recommend using a bit of restraint and a bunch of self-awareness. If you listen closely, you will hear your body talking to you. That's the goal throughout this entire journey— listen to your body and obey what it's telling you. If something doesn't feel good, don't do it.

"I Don't Feel Like It" Days

Okay! Don't do it. Whatever IT is. It's more than okay to take some days off to do absolutely nothing productive at all. But when you feel better, you should do better. And if you don't feel like going to your favorite Tai Chi class, maybe you could do a few moves in your living room or stretch in bed. Again. SOMETHING is usually better than NOTHING. But you are the boss of yourself. Just try not to let too many "I don't feel like it" days add up in a row.

It's also critical that you recognize the difference between depression and actual illness. Sickness is a top-notch reason to stay in bed. The opposite is true for depression. When cancer gets you "down in the dumps", isolating yourself in bed will only further those bad feelings. If you identify that your bad feelings are more emotional than physical, force yourself up and out for some movement and fresh air. Music and camaraderie might help as well. You can incorporate the outdoors, uplifting music, and family and friends during your workouts to improve your mental health along the way.

Managing the Opinions of Others

Friends and family who think it's outrageous for you to even consider exercising during cancer treatment may be discouraging. That's common. However, your responsibility is to yourself and your health, and hopefully, you now understand the value of fitness to your comeback. I recommend expressing your appreciation for their concern. Follow up by encouraging them to check out the endless amounts of research proving cancer patients benefit from exercise and quality nutrition. Inform them that you're concerned about becoming too weak and immobile, losing strength and balance. The stronger and fitter you are, the less fragile you'll be and the more quickly you will bounce back. You can say "Fitz Koehler, says …" but it'll probably sound best coming straight from you.

CHAPTER FIVE

NeWLy DiaGNoSeD

Simply stated, the stronger and healthier you are going into any sort of physical crisis, the easier it will be to rebound and recover. If you have been committed to a healthy body pre-diagnosis, it's a great time to pat yourself on the back. That won't guarantee any of this will be easy, but it will certainly make things less difficult and potentially allow you to avoid many pitfalls. However, if you haven't been on top of your health leading into this insanity, you are where you are and neither one of us has a time machine. The great news though, is that there may still be time for you to improve your situation before you begin your treatments. Many people have weeks or months between diagnosis and the start of care. If you're one of those people, you should make good use of that time.

Consider the Four Pillars of Fitness and put in some time daily to improve at each. Start wherever you are with your capabilities and take baby steps toward improvements. Cancer is terrifying and comes with exorbitant amounts of emotional strain. Even though I'm known to be a "tough cookie," I often sat alone in my car sobbing. Exercise helped me manage those ugly feelings that cancer treatment often brings. Vigorous cardio and strength training enabled me to vent much of the toxic anguish pent up inside me which was very relieving. I would walk into the gym with a cranky face and walk out with a far more positive outlook. I did my best to stay in constant motion during the days before I began treatment.

Medical appointments may make your schedule look strange, but if you plan wisely and aggressively, you can squeeze both large and small amounts of exercise in. Laser focus on being active and improving physically no matter what. If you're always working to do better and be better, you will make progress, it's inevitable. And when it comes to thriving during cancer care, these efforts will, at the very minimum, slow your decline. Stronger is always better than weaker! Better balance is always better than being unsteady. Being mobile is better than being tight and inflexible. Having stamina is better than being easily winded. These might be considered obvious statements, but unless you're consistently fighting for your health, it can easily slip away. Your commitment to moving your body in challenging ways whenever possible will make your survival experience infinitely better.

Scheduling Exercise:

If your schedule is flexible and uncomplicated, plan workouts as you normally would. No biggie. Just do it.

- Run
- Cycle
- Swim
- Box
- Take Group Fitness Classes
- Strength Train
- Do Yoga
- Play Sports
- Hike
- Anything else you like to do!

If your schedule is challenging, plan for a few shorter workouts like these that require little to no preparation.

- Go for a vigorous walk alone, with friends, or with the dog.
- Start and end each day with, at minimum, short walks.
- Take a short fitness class or follow along with workout videos on the internet. They can be free, convenient, and won't require travel or prep time.
- Do a quick circuit at your desk at work or out in your backyard. Choose five exercises. Do one, two, or three sets of each. For example Jumping Jacks, squats, push-ups, lunges, and dips. Repeat!
- Play upbeat music in your house and shake your thang.
- Get outside and play ball with your people.
- Chase your dog around the couch.
- Wrestle with your kids or spouse.

If your schedule is packed, plan to squeeze in brief activities in weird places.

- Walk laps around the medical plaza or through the hospital corridors.
- While waiting in exam rooms: march in place, jump, do jumping jacks, do pushups against the wall, dips off the side of the exam table, lunges, squats, or stretch. Just don't do anything which requires touching the floor. I imagine they're semi-gross.
- Stretch in the shower.
- Calf raises or stretches while you wait in lines.
- Stand on one foot to improve balance while waiting in lines.

Newly Diagnosed Nutrition

This is the perfect time to meet with a registered dietitian. No, not the personal trainer at your gym or the random neighbor who sells weight loss shakes and other snake oil products. Definitely not your friend with the most fabulous body. You should specifically connect with a registered dietitian who has expertise in consulting with cancer patients. Your oncologist will more than likely have several recommendations for you. Food is an essential tool for health in any circumstance. Eating wisely for nourishment during cancer care is paramount to your success. Not only are you going to want to know which nutrients will help strengthen your body's ability to fight your disease, but you'll want to know what to avoid. You may also experience food sensitivities, suffer from a volatile stomach, lose your sense of taste, and/or have surgeries that restrict your eating habits. It's tricky! My cancer was only in my breast and adjacent lymph nodes, it hadn't even come close to my digestive system. Nevertheless, chemo wreaked havoc on my innards and eating/drinking became incredibly complicated. As many patients do, I lost about 10-percent of my body weight which put me in the "scrawny" verging on "emaciated" category. A reminder that not all weight loss is a good thing. I was able to stall the loss before it became a huge obstacle, but that's only because I got aggressive with nutrition. On the flip side, many patients gain lots of weight during treatment because of stress, inactivity, overeating, and the effects of pharmaceuticals. We will talk more about the power of nutrition in Chapter 8, but I want you to seek guidance from a credentialed expert and continue the conversation as your treatment progresses. Do not ignore this step. It will pay off!

Treatment Begins

Whether you start with chemotherapy, radiation, or surgery, the way your body responds is a crapshoot. While it's important to continue living while working to save your life, it might also be wise to dial your workouts back as you tread into unchartered territories. The ramifications of each type of treatment along with the specifics of your case will vary. Hopefully, these next few suggestions will help you manage each step successfully.

Staying Healthy After Surgery

Having surgery tends to require a certain amount of rest and recovery time, which often comes with very clear or strict doctor's orders on what you can and cannot do. Yielding to that guidance is a wise way to avoid unnecessary setbacks. If your surgeon says not to lift anything over 10 pounds for two weeks, you simply need to do what you're told. Even if you feel strong like Superman. Risking regression, re-opening of your wound, strains, falls or worse would just be foolish. Once you've chosen a surgeon you trust and have allowed him or her to reorganize your innards, trust that the follow-up advice will be solid as well.

The reality is that most doctors want you to move and be active. They know how harmful a sedentary lifestyle can be. They also have a deep understanding of your trauma and know what it will take for you to recoup. In most circumstances, as soon as they believe movement will do more good than harm, they will encourage you to get up and get going. Quite often, they will start the process with a prescription for physical therapy. If yours does not, you should inquire about it. Why? Physical therapists specialize in helping damaged, weak, and stiff people build the strength, stamina, mobility, and balance necessary to return to normal activities. They will do a precise evaluation of your body and analyze exactly what needs to be done to solve your problems. Combining exercises and a variety of therapeutic modalities, they can often work miracles. I've utilized physical therapy to recover from a variety of issues throughout my life with great success. The PT I saw throughout my cancer care was worth his weight in gold. He helped me regain mobility while reducing pain and breaking up scar tissue.

You may see a PT before you leave the hospital, one may come to your home, or you may have to venture to an office once or multiple times a week. Given the opportunity, I'd recommend taking it. If it's affordable, keep going until the PT purposely releases you from treatment. The benefits will keep coming if you show up and do what you're told. And if you do get released from PT, continue doing the exercises prescribed at home. When you stop doing them, you will likely experience some regression.

It's also important to recognize that you may only need to rest a body part, not your entire body. For example, if you've had surgery on your breasts, there may be no reason to prevent your lower body from walking, lunging, squatting, or pedaling.

Ostomies, Incisions, and Rashes ... Oh my!

If you have open wounds, recent incisions, an ostomy, burns, rashes, or any sort of issue which might make certain exercises complicated, please reach out to your medical team for guidance. You can be confident that oodles of people before you have confronted the same or similar obstacles and there's a great chance one of your practitioners has a simple solution for you. Don't be shy! Always ask for guidance when you need some. Instead of worrying about being a bother, your enthusiasm for health and fitness might impress your team and put happy smiles on their faces. Sometimes medical procedures stop us completely. Sometimes they only force us to be creative!

Staying Healthy During Chemotherapy

The start of chemotherapy is a really good time to purposefully slow your roll since the drugs will affect your entire system. At least for a while. Some patients instantly feel the effects of nausea, fatigue, dizziness, dehydration, etc. Some patients never experience anything of the sort. Many of us respond a few days after chemo or even after a few weeks. So, this curious experience is one you should manage as you go, with baby steps being the game plan.

If you feel great in the immediate hours and days after an infusion, feel free to go for a walk or do other gentle exercises. However, I would not plan for a 10-mile run the day after chemo. That would be ambitious and super cool if you did it without consequence. However, if you push yourself too hard while your body is hosting the world's weirdest science experiment, you might have some regrets. Chemo can induce both mental fog and dehydration, amongst other issues. Do NOT pursue exercises that require tremendous focus or balance. Instead, work at a low level, ideally in comfortable temperatures. Exercising outdoors mid-summer when the temperatures are in the high 80s isn't wise – unless you're in the water. Choose wisely. And stay near folks who care for you, just in case you need some support.

Unlike with surgery, you probably won't walk out of chemo with strict rules for lifting, reaching, and jumping. Plan to be gentle with yourself and only move in a way that feels completely comfortable. This is not the time to attempt gains with your lifting or increase the pace at which you ride your bike. You are going to have to self-monitor and make cautious decisions as you go.

Staying hydrated is always important, but even more so now. Dehydration can lead to extreme fatigue, dizziness, loss of balance, and falls. A volatile stomach will definitely increase these symptoms. Friend, they have pumped you full of helpful but nasty drugs. You must drink water. Chemo plus exercise-induced dehydration is a recipe for disaster. Be smart. Keep a water bottle with you at all times and drink from it.

Exercising During Radiation

Much like the other forms of cancer treatments, exercising during radiation therapy can ease side effects, including fatigue, anemia, and sleeplessness. Depending on which body part you are having zapped, your doctor may or may not give strict recommendations on exercises to avoid.

Make it a point to ask for guidance. When I had radiation, I discovered that it was not advised to swim because the chlorine could dry out my skin making me more susceptible to burns. I asked my radiology oncologist about it and she confirmed that it might be better for me to put swimming on hold until I was done with that portion of my care. Your doctor may not feel the same way. So, ask! Also, if balance becomes an issue, stick with seated exercises or those you can do lying down.

Prioritizing Sleep

Quality sleep is vital to health because it is the time when your body and brain recover from previous stressors and recharge for the next. Seven hours is recommended for healthy adults, but cancer patients may require more. Consider it part of your efforts to heal. Treatment, stress, and pharmaceuticals can increase fatigue which makes it harder to focus, exercise, maintain a healthy weight, and fight off illness. Your body needs as much revitalizing rest as possible.

Go to bed at a reasonable hour each night and sleep in a bit whenever you need. Build naps into your schedule as well. It's not lazy to snooze during the day when you're battling cancer. It's brilliant. Thirty-minute power naps can go a long way to help you get through your days, and if you need to nap longer, do so! Lastly, if you're suffering from insomnia, don't hesitate to speak to your doctor.

Spend some effort making your bedroom conducive to quality sleep. Remove the clutter, and invest in blankets, comforters, and pillows that feel luxurious. You can find quality bedding at an affordable price. Set up a fan bedside to instantly respond to hot flashes or chills. It will also provide some "white noise", to help you rest when your family, roomies, or neighbors are being loud, especially during the day when you might want to take a nap. Lastly, if you tend to watch TV as you doze off, set the sleep timer so it automatically turns off within an hour and won't disrupt your quality of sleep throughout the night.

No matter which segment of cancer care you're embarking on, you are going to have to blend commitment, enthusiasm, and caution. I encourage you to maintain your focus on health and fitness while listening to both your doctors and your body. Remain optimistic that exercise will be a highlight of your days.

CHAPTER SIX

SiCK to StRoNG

If you're looking in the mirror thinking "what happened to me?" don't worry, there is hope. Think about the incredible recoveries you've seen from people who were in traumatic accidents. Car crashes, sports injuries, and fires. The human body is an extraordinary organism with almost magical abilities to rebuild and recover. For that to occur though, you're going to have to put in the work. Smart, strategic, relentless work. I believe in you. I hope you do too.

I often reflect on my experience with cancer and laugh at the fact that my cancerous tumor and lymph nodes never actually caused me any pain, suffering, or sickness. I felt fabulous before I started treatment. My 15 months' worth of chemo, radiation and surgeries did their job of beating the heck out of my cancer cells, which was fantastic, but they also beat the heck out of me. Ironic, but worth it. Of course, many people are sickened and struggle because of their actual disease. It seems no one gets out unscathed. Just remember that exercise and quality nutrition will help your normal cells survive treatment better and recover quicker. It will also make your body a more hostile environment for those cancer cells!

Start where you are.

Instead of comparing yourself to the way you used to be or the capabilities that you used to have, accept where you are today and do one thing that will help you become better. When I started to feel relief from intense sickness, my first move was to get into my neighborhood pool and wiggle. I kid you not. I didn't even consider walking or swimming in that pool. I literally just stood in the shallow end and wiggled. Talk about refreshing! It was the perfect, non-threatening start of my journey back to being super fit. My next few visits to the pool included more wiggling, some stretching, and eventually, water walking. Swimming started a couple of weeks later. Instead of getting overzealous when my efforts felt good, I progressed as slowly as I could to avoid setbacks. This method of avoiding setbacks at all costs was wildly successful for me. That's what I'm hoping for you as well.

Baby steps for the win!

You must commit to wisely making progress without doing any harm. If you do too much too soon, you'll likely experience an uncomfortable setback which is the last thing you need. Start at a pace or level you think is ridiculously easy, leisurely, and enjoyable, and then increase your frequency, intensity, and time in tiny increments. You should also vary the type of exercise you do. You will NOT regret avoiding self-induced suffering. And you'll have the rest of your life to achieve beast mode if that's on your wish list.

Maintain a healthy mindset!

Walking back into a fitness studio or gym after being whacked by cancer can be emotionally exhausting. Because you're not what you used to be, you may look at your diminished physique and capabilities and feel intimidated or embarrassed. Don't! After my mean chemo prevented me from exercising in the gym for three entire months, I finally ventured back. When I sat down to use a strength training machine and found I could only lift about 20-percent of the weight I used to, I felt shame and disappointment. This is same shame millions of people experience who fear they don't fit in at a fitness center. But then I reminded myself of the things I've been impressing upon others for decades.

1. Everyone who steps foot in a fitness facility to exercise is a winner. I mean it. If you show up to better yourself, I admire you, and you should be proud.

2. Nobody else cares about what you're doing! They're all too busy worrying about their own workouts and the way they look to be concerned with what YOU are doing. Think about when you're in the gym— are you really concerned about how other people look?

Who in the world had any clue what weight I used to lift and knew that I was lifting less? How self-involved could I be to imagine they would? So I didn't. Instead, I chose to be:

- Proud of myself for showing up.
- Grateful that I was back in a gym.
- Enthusiastic about making my physical comeback.

This clarity was a real bonus as I puttered along making little bits of progress. And the reality was, if anyone was checking me out, it was probably because of my beautiful bald head. You are under strict orders to remain positive and hold your head up high whenever you exercise. You are a person on a mission and that is to be celebrated! This is also the time to show some real compassion for yourself. You've suffered too much to punish yourself with foolish mental games. So don't. Choose pride instead.

Set goals.

It's critical to know where you are going before you try and map out a plan to get there. Get where? Only you can answer the question: Whom do you want to be? Throughout my career, it has been the first thing I've asked people who've come to me for guidance. I can only share effective advice once I've been informed of a person's vision for themselves. How do you want your body to feel, perform and look? Are symmetry, balance, mobility, and strength important to you? Would you like to build back enough endurance to walk through a mall, outdoor festival, or theme park? Would you like to touch your toes with your legs straight, or be able to stand up after being seated on the ground without using your hands? Would you like to gain or lose weight? Do you want to play sports, for leisure or for competition? Perhaps a marathon or triathlon is in your future. Would you like to be able to do more, feel more powerful, and look even fitter than you did before cancer? These are all wonderful ideas, but your destination is completely up to you. Think about your priorities and write them down in your *Healthy Cancer Comeback Journal* or in the notes app on your phone. Update your goals as you make progress. Each milestone accomplished, no matter how little, is worth celebrating! Whether you've increased the weights you lift by 1 pound or shortened your mile time by 2 minutes, always pat yourself on the back for any amount of progress.

Chemo Butt.

I hope you've figured out by now that this book is not about vanity. However, it's definitely okay to care about the way your body looks and to work to achieve certain standards. I wrote about "chemo butt" in my memoir *My Noisy Cancer Comeback: Running at the Mouth, While Running for My Life*, and I think it's worth mentioning here as well. "Chemo butt" was the name I gave to the saggy flat pancake that replaced my once plump and firm tush. After losing fourteen pounds of mostly muscle, I was horrified when I caught a glimpse of my derriere, which now looked like it belonged to someone in their nineties. I did not enjoy that experience at all. But I did like the spark it lit inside me and the pleasure I took rebuilding my booty. My overall fit appearance certainly suffered as all of my muscles atrophied, but rebuilding my backside became symbolic of my zealous quest for fitness. Every other day I performed a wide variety of squats, lunges, leg presses, and lateral movements with bands. Over time, I was delighted by even the smallest bits of visible progress and thrilled when my flat pancake had blossomed back into a plum. Chemo butt was not cool, but restoring the junk in my trunk, as well as all of my other muscles, has been a real source of pride. It's okay if you look forward to that too.

Aging and Cancer

It's important to recognize that many cancer patients are in their golden years and may no longer be interested in athletic adventures. Without discouraging anyone from seeking out big challenges, if that's no longer your calling, please pursue a fit body to maintain the quality of your life. Preventing falls should be a top priority, as more than 25% of adults over 65 take a spill each year.[4] These falls are responsible for pain, disability, loss of independence, and premature death. Strength and balance training are powerful weapons against falls. You'll also benefit from disrupting common aging burdens like arthritis, muscle atrophy, stiffness and weakness-induced pain. Fit seniors are more likely to be able to shop, cook, clean, enjoy quality time with family (grandchildren perhaps), travel, drive and maintain their independence. From your first day until your final day, your health always matters. Choose exercises you can do to keep your body mobile, strong and flexible.

WAGING YOUR COMEBACK

Extremely Weak or New to Exercise
- Start with a couple of minutes of Level I exercises.
- Move for 10 minutes or less.
- Your goal here is to get your body reacquainted with movement. Do not push too hard, move too much, or do anything that feels remotely

uncomfortable.
- You should experience delight with the simple act of deliberately being in motion.

Less Weak
- Blend Level 1 and 2 exercises as you see fit.
- Aim for multiple 10-minute exercise sessions
- Build up to 20 minutes at a time.
- Engaging in activities that look a little more like standard exercise should build your confidence.

Feeling Decent
- Blend Level 2 and 3 exercises as you see fit.
- Instead of finding one exercise you love and sticking with it, force yourself to branch out. Your body will benefit from moving in a variety of ways.
- Maintain control of your pace and your commitment to baby steps.

Fit and Athletic
- Blend Level 2-4 exercises as you see fit.
- Challenge your body in ways that make you huff and puff, grunt, wince, and wobble.
- Choose an athletic goal to achieve and create/find a plan to help you get there.
- Return to sports and competition.
- Pursue exciting and elevated goals for yourself.

Exercise Rules

If you're in crisis, rest. You can gently stretch, but don't push your body to do more than just recover.

If you're not in crisis but don't feel fantastic, pursue mobility and light activities. Little things like walking to the mailbox, or doing a few stretches and strength training moves with resistance bands will minimize stiffness and soreness.

If you feel decent, do some activities or exercises that feel good without exhausting you.

If you feel great, pursue enhanced fitness with vigor.

Level 1 Exercises

- Walk around your house or hospital floor
- Walk to the mailbox
- Stand up and sit down in your chair multiple times
- Slow walk or hike
- Wiggle around in the water
- Water Walking
- Stretches in pool
- Stretches in bed
- Super slow pedaling on a recumbent stationary bike
- Chair exercises without added resistance
- Light strength training with your own body weight
- Balance training

Level 2 Exercises at Low Intensity

- Walk or hike outside
- Visit a zoo
- Walk through the mall or in a large store for temperature controlled environment
- Cardio equipment at an easy level
- Water walk
- Swim leisurely
- Water fitness class

- Aqua Therapy
- Casual cycling
- Play Ping Pong
- Tai Chi
- Serve tennis balls- don't chase them!
- Light strength training with your own body weight, light dumbbells, or resistance bands
- Slow dance
- Chair fitness
- Frisbee
- Canoe with partner
- Play catch
- Pilates
- Yoga
- Golf - driving range
- Mini golf
- Balance training

Level 3 Exercises at Moderate Pace

- Walk or hike
- Swim laps
- Water fitness class
- Cycle
- Canoe
- Stand-up Paddleboarding
- Surf
- Ski (water or snow)
- Wake Board
- Snow Board
- Play golf
- Shoot hoops (with or without running around)
- Doubles tennis

- Volleyball
- Kick a ball
- Play catch
- Dance fitness
- Group fitness classes
- Cardio equipment up to a medium level
- Pilates
- Yoga
- Martial arts
- Tennis
- Racquetball
- Pickleball
- Run for short bursts of time at a slow-moderate pace
- Balance training

Level 4 Exercises

Start working toward higher intensity and challenging yourself.

- Walk or hike at a fast pace
- Run
- Cycle
- Canoe
- Stand Up Paddleboard
- Dance
- Cardio equipment up to an advanced level
- Advanced group fitness classes
- Boot camp
- Triathlon
- Functional fitness classes
- Pilates
- Yoga
- Snowshoe
- Climb stadium steps

- Martial arts
- Mountain Climbing
- Boxing
- Soccer
- All Sports
- Balance training

Elite Fitness and Athleticism

Once you move past your cancer-induced bubble of vulnerability, the prospects of becoming very fit and athletic can become quite exciting. If you've earned the status of feeling somewhat "normal", I encourage you to seriously invest in becoming the best new version of yourself. Cancer tried to stop you, and it couldn't. So use that momentum to live your life to the fullest in a body you feel fantastic about. This is the time to start working with fewer restraints. You are not being poisoned by chemo, zapped by radiation, or healing from surgeries. You are no longer dealing with acute side effects. Push the envelope and train vigorously!

My guidance for the general population (welcome back to it) is as follows:

- Maintain perspective and stay positive. Your body needs compassion and enthusiasm.
- Decide who you want to be. Make a list of very specific goals. It's not only okay, but ideal to be ambitious. Aim high and continually celebrate your progress!
- Detail activities you'd like to be able to perform, and how you'd like your body to feel and look.
- Create a plan including all Four Pillars of Fitness.
- Choose an athletic goal and sign up for it.
- Exercise most days of the week.

- Challenge yourself with each workout. You should be huffing and puffing, grunting, wincing, and wobbling!
- Aim to smell bad and look awful by the end of your workouts. Drenched with sweat, stinky and rosy red are good things in fitness.
- Gradually increase the amount of time you put into each workout.
- Diversify your workouts to prevent them from becoming monotonous, and to challenge your body in a variety of ways.
- Utilize the power of nutrition to help you reach your goals, along with the Exact Formula to reach and maintain your goal weight.

Choosing a lofty goal is going to be the compass that steers you in the right direction, and signing up for an event will have a strong impact on your focus and determination. Commit to something bold. I'll share that four weeks after my 21st and final round of chemo, I participated in a Spartan 5K obstacle course race. I went pretty darn slow and failed on a bunch of the strength-oriented challenges. But I laughed far more than anyone else, delighted in being covered in mud, and took enormous pride in crossing the finish line. Filthy, happy, and proud, nobody enjoyed their athletic adventure more than I did that day.

A week after this Spartan 5K, I ambitiously showed up for a mini-sprint triathlon. This event included 100 yards of swimming in a lake, 11 miles of cycling around the lake, and two miles on foot. I couldn't have been more elated to start as I stood lakeside in my swimsuit and cap. From there, I proceeded to finish the swim last, behind pregnant women, children, and elderly people. I then got on my bike to go further than I'd ever ridden before. My legs were burning by mile eight, but when I hit the steep long hill before the finish line I had to dismount. I was hyperventilating and simply couldn't pedal forward without pausing to catch my breath. There I stood, in the middle of the road as a police car with flashing lights trailed behind me (a safety measure to make sure the final athlete returns safely). Perspective mandated that I could only think about how fortunate I was to be doing THIS particular hard thing as opposed to the way more horrible hard thing I was doing one year prior (chemo). To me, exercise-induced suffering was way more fun and interesting than being beaten up by cancer. In fact, thinking back to how sick and weak I was and realizing how far I'd come filled me with adrenaline. I finished that triathlon with a combination of walking and running and the pride of an Olympic gold medalist. Yay me! I am not promoting stepping wildly outside of your abilities or being reckless. I was fully aware of my capabilities, and even though I struggled, I paced myself well. However, I absolutely do not want you to fear hard work, physical challenges, or even failure. If I hadn't finished that race, who would've cared? I might have been slightly disappointed, but I also would have acknowledged how badass it was for me to try! I was in a win-win situation.

About a year later I was personally invited to run the Boston Marathon by a charity. I'd never run more than a half marathon (13.1 miles) previously and spent the night going back and forth over whether I'd accept. 24 hours later, after considering what cancer had put me through, I thought … comparatively, how hard could a marathon be? So I set off on my training program and conquered that 26.2-miler four months later. Was the Boston Marathon tough? Sure! Did I ever think "gee I wish I hadn't agreed to do this?" Not once. In fact, with every step, I felt elation because I was living boldly. Not only had I conquered a terrifying bout with cancer, but I was once again strong and athletic!

So what will YOU do to make all of your days count? What will you choose as a platform for building your body back better than ever? I hope that you find something that seems both enjoyable and challenging. Once you've

Sample Fitness Goals

- Run/walk any distance race
- Complete a triathlon, cycling event, or obstacle course race
- Swim for competition
- Earn a black belt in a form of martial arts
- Take a dance class and perform in a show
- Hike a challenging trail
- Climb a mountain
- Learn a new water sport: skiing, surfing, wakeboarding
- Learn a new snow sport: skiing, snowboarding, cross country skiing
- Do a certain amount of push-ups or pull-ups
- Compete in a full season of tennis, softball, kickball, flag football, or pickleball

For endurance racing, start with short distance events and gradually progress to longer distances.

Keep track of your progress, set goals, and record memories with the *Healthy Cancer Comeback Journal!*

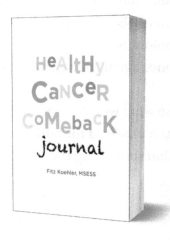

CHAPTER SEVEN

EVERYTHING EXERCISE

When you know better, you do better.

Strength Training - What You Should Know

I'm going to kick this conversation off with a question for those who have shied away from strength training in the past. On any given day doing any given thing, would you rather be stronger or weaker? Can you come up with one single instance when weakness is superior to strength? I'm confident you'll come to the conclusion that strength is always superior. If you have believed that strength training would make you bulky, you were wrong. Even for men, bulky muscles take a lot of effort and usually only come to those who are working extremely hard and fueling them aggressively with food. Women often fear that strength training will make them "big" which is quite sad, because, for the most part, women do not make enough testosterone to generate excessive muscle mass. Certainly not muscles that would be considered "bulky." One might be surprised to know that strength training actually boosts your metabolism and can enhance your weight loss efforts. Another consequence of skipping strength training for women is an increased susceptibility for osteoporosis, as it is vital for building bone density. For your healthy cancer comeback, it's important to focus on the power and capabilities strength training will yield.

All of your muscles matter. That's right. All of them! Strength training isn't just about big biceps and flat abdominal muscles. Strength training is about having the ability to move your body in a variety of ways, with the power to pull, push, lift, and press against resistance. It's about being able to hoist yourself off of the ground with ease, as well as carry groceries into your home without struggle. Strength is required to open that jar of pickles, slam your car's trunk shut, and hold your grandchild. Your back, lats, shoulders, and glutes are challenged regularly by even the most mundane tasks, so it would be unacceptable to ignore them when you exercise.

It's also important to mention that many people tend to work what I call "vanity muscles," and neglect the others. Strong curvy biceps, abs, and glutes are always popular, but training only the muscles you enjoy checking out in the mirror would be foolish. Now that cancer threatens to weaken you, it's time to fight back by building and maintaining strength across your entire body. I assure you, weakness has no benefits.

We discussed the F.I.T.T. Principle in Chapter 3, but there are a few things particular to strength training you should know. And a quick reminder that to make progress, strength training should make you grunt.

The 48-Hour Rule. Studies show that to reap the benefits of strength training, your muscles need approximately 48 hours to rest, recover, and rebuild between workouts. Effective strength training actually causes tiny tears in your muscle fibers. These are good tears, which your body will remedy with its fancy response team. These tears are the reason your muscles feel so sore and weak after a workout. However, if you do not allow a 48-hour window for your muscle repair to take place, then your muscles remain in a constant state of breakdown. So, if you work your biceps on

Monday morning, just wait until Wednesday morning to train them again. This rule is relevant to all of your muscles, including your abs. It is also exclusive to strength training.

Opposing Muscle Groups. Opposing muscles are those that work against each other. Ideally, these muscles will possess equal strength. Your biceps, for example, are responsible for bending your arms while your triceps do the work of extending your arms. If your biceps are significantly stronger than your triceps, you risk injury to the weaker triceps and your elbow joint. I advise putting an equal amount of effort into training both. If you can lift 15 pounds doing a biceps curl, you should be able to press 15 pounds for a triceps extension.

Other opposing muscle groups:

- Back (traps) vs Chest (pecs)
- Shoulders (deltoids) vs Lats
- Biceps vs Triceps
- Quadriceps vs Hamstrings
- Calves vs Anterior Tibialis
- Abductors vs Adductors
- Abdominals vs Low Back (Erector Spinae)
- Iliopsoas vs Glutes

Train larger muscles first.

It's a wise idea to start working your largest muscles which are closest to your belly button first. This is because we usually need our smaller muscles (accessory muscles) to help activate and work our larger muscles. But we do not necessarily need our larger muscles to work our smaller muscles. If, for example, you did some killer exercises that fatigued your biceps and triceps, those smaller muscles would not likely be able to perform well enough to do chest-focused exercises such as the bench press or push-ups. You need your arms to work your chest. However, you do not need to activate your chest muscles to work your arms. So, split your body in half and make sure you target the largest muscles first. Quick tip: your larger muscles are closest to your belly button. Start close to it and work your way out toward your fingers and toes.

Sample order for an upper body strength training session:

- Chest
- Back
- Shoulders
- Lats
- Biceps
- Triceps
- Forearms

Sample order for a lower body strength training session:

- Glutes
- Hip flexors
- Quadriceps
- Hamstrings
- Adductors
- Abductors
- Anterior Tibialis
- Calves

Core training comes last!

Since your abdominal and lower back muscles must be strong to help maintain proper form for most exercises, train them last. If you train them before exercises like push-ups or military presses, your form could suffer putting you at risk for pain or injury.

How to choose the perfect amount of resistance.

Your priority is to find a resistance that challenges you without hurting you. Whether you are utilizing dumbbells, kettlebells, machines, bands, your body weight, or any other strength training tool, figuring out how much will only come via trial and error. Always start with a choice you believe will be easy and advance in small increments as you feel comfortable. Choose a resistance that forces you to grunt by the eighth repetition. If you can't do at least six reps of your exercise, you should reduce the resistance. If you can easily do far more than 10 repetitions, you should try a heavier option. If you are struggling to lift your arms and legs, or stand up without any additional tools, that's okay too. Sometimes gravity is all the resistance you need, especially if cancer has beat you up. If this is true for you, be compassionate with yourself! Consider your limbs your dumbbells and get serious about lifting them in all directions to get stronger. Every exercise I recommend with equipment can be done without. Stay consistent and you'll be working with resistance tools soon enough.

How many repetitions should you do?

Welp, that answer varies as well. If you're just getting started, aim to do 10 repetitions of a weight that feels mildly challenging. Work your way up to three sets of 10 repetitions over time. Your goal should be to choose enough resistance that reps 8-10 always feel like a struggle and make you grunt. If you are working toward putting on serious size and strength, choose the type of resistance that will exhaust your muscles in 6-8 reps. More weight + fewer reps = bigger stronger muscles.

"What if I only want to tone?"

That's a common question I'm asked, and here's my honest answer. There is no such thing as toning. Either you are working to grow stronger or you aren't. "Toning" is often the wish of women who fear bulkiness. Remember, unless you're using steroids or making massive efforts to grow large muscles, you won't. I'm looking you in the eyes right now. Strength training will only make you better. Do not skip this pillar!

Cool Strength Training Tools:

- Your body may be your best tool because you never have to pay to use your body, you always have it with you and you only need gravity to have a challenging workout.
- Dumbbells are probably the most popular strength training tool, popular at fitness centers and for home use. They come in tons of different sizes, and can be used sitting, standing, or laying down.
- Resistance Bands are very inexpensive and can be used to work most muscle groups. They're gentle yet challenging and are often a preferred choice for injured people rehabbing in physical therapy and body builders alike. They are lightweight and easy to travel with.
- Cable Machines are larger machines that allow you to do similar exercises as you do with bands, with the ability to add resistance.
- Kettlebells are relatively small pieces of equipment that work your muscles in a wide range of motion and are fun to use.
- Machines are most commonly found at fitness centers. They are large and provide a stable choice for working one muscle at a time, often without having to utilize your core for stability. Machines make it easy to adjust resistance, and often come with instructions posted on them.

Cardio - What You Should Know

The main intention of cardiovascular exercise, also known as cardiorespiratory exercise, is to increase the capacity and strength of your heart and lungs. The more powerful your heart is, the more easily it will pump oxygen-rich blood through your body. This lowers your heart rate and blood pressure which are symbolic of good health and fitness. Increasing your lung capacity strengthens your breathing muscles making it easier to deliver oxygen to your body and brain. The stronger your heart and lungs are, the more comfortable vigorous exercise will be, and the longer it will take your body to exhaust or "poop out."

In the second paragraph of this book, I mentioned a phenomenal 2022 study from Tel Aviv University that found that high-intensity aerobic exercise can reduce the risk of metastatic cancer by 72-percent. Professor Carmit Levy and Dr. Ytach Gepner say that intense aerobic exercise increases the glucose (sugar) consumption of internal organs, thereby reducing energy availability to the tumor. "If the general message to the public so far has been 'be active, be healthy'," they say, "now we can explain how aerobic activity can maximize the prevention of the most aggressive and metastatic types of cancer." This is precisely the type of control we've been discussing in this book. Exercise is a powerful weapon against cancer, and this information should inspire even the laziest people to spring into action. As the sweat drips off of you, raise an evil eyebrow and shout, "starve, cancer cells, starve!"

Vigorous is a subjective term depending on who is doing the work. Anything that makes YOU huff and puff for an extended period should be considered vigorous. Do not compare yourself to anyone else. If walking down the hall in the hospital today makes you huff and puff, we are going to consider it your vigorous cardio. Today's efforts should make tomorrow's easier, and constant efforts will eventually make today's struggles look like child's play.

Progress will reveal itself when you can do things comfortably that previously made you huff and puff. This is what stamina and endurance look like. Continuous efforts to do a little more and a little more will turn your fatigue into fitness and if you keep going, athleticism. Additionally, cardio is a superb choice for burning calories.

While getting your heart rate up with vigorous exercise for even a tiny burst of time is beneficial, the gold standard for cardio would be doing at least 30 minutes daily. If you've got 10 or 20 minutes, go for it. If you can do two-three hours of cardio, even better yet!

But let's come back to earth. If cancer has kicked your booty, skip the gold standard and stick with YOUR standard! Start with one minute at a time. One minute of walking, wiggling, swimming, or dancing once or a few times a day can be your starting point. Increase your cardio to two minutes, three, five, and so on. You've got to start somewhere, and right now, you can only start where you are.

Cardio - Moves to Make You Huff and Puff

- Cycling stationery or on the road
- Walking
- Hiking
- Running
- Group fitness classes
- Swimming
- Aqua walking jogging
- Dance - all sorts
- Martial arts
- Canoeing
- Stand Up Paddleboarding
- Snow Shoeing
- Cardio machines such as elliptical

- Basketball
- Soccer
- Lacrosse
- Ultimate Frisbee

Stretching - What You Should Know

Keeping your muscles flexible and your body mobile are some of the most significant things you can do to avoid pain, and genuinely feel good. Does anyone say "My back is so stiff," with a positive connotation? Never. This is why a consistent effort to keep your muscles pliable is so valuable. Your joints will also benefit from stretching. Remember that your arms should be able to go through an enormous circular range of motion from your shoulder joint. To maintain that range, you should perform that motion daily. The same goes for your hips and spine. Humans were not built to move only in a linear forward motion (walking, sitting, lying flat). Instead, we were designed to rotate, twist, move laterally, and bend. Stretching is the perfect time to put your joints and muscles through their complete ranges of motion. As the old saying goes, "if you don't use it, you lose it." Avoid unnecessary pain and discomfort by simply bending, reaching, and twisting a bunch. And just like strength training, you should stretch all of your muscles. Not just your hamstrings.

Stretching at the end of a workout session is the ideal time to make progress with flexibility. Once your core temperature has increased and your body has performed a variety of motions, your muscles are ripe for progress. The ending of a workout is a good time to stretch until you wince. Hold each stretch for 10-20 seconds. Relax for a few moments, and repeat.

Taking a lengthy stretching or yoga class is a superb idea, but stretching can and should be done throughout your day with any amount being beneficial. I highly recommend stretching in bed before you get up and before you go to sleep. You can also stretch in bed when you're stuck there not feeling so good. Stretch in the shower, at your desk, in the exam room while you wait for your doctor, at the park while your kids play, or in the airport bathroom between flights. There is no wrong place or time to stretch.

If flexibility is a high priority, pursue yoga or Tai Chi. Look online to find free classes on the internet, or find a studio nearby to take part in a group or do personal training.

Warning! While Hot Yoga has many benefits for the average bloke, doing it during cancer care may be unwise. The heat may be harmful for those enduring or recovering from chemo, radiation, surgeries and/or other pharmaceuticals. Please check with your doctor before you pursue hot yoga.

Balance Training - What You Should Know

If you don't like falling, this should be high on your list of priorities. Remember that even the most impressive athletes sometimes take a tumble and without exception, they wish they hadn't. To make progress in balance training, you should always be testing it. And by testing it I mean that you should do things that make you wobble, adjust and look like you are off-balance. If you are standing on one foot motionless, you are not making progress. If you are standing on one foot flailing your arms around like a drunk … you are doing the right thing. As with the other three Pillars of Fitness, struggle leads to progress.

Balance training will usually require you to stand on one foot, stand on something squishy, or both. If you're super unsteady, try standing on one foot while holding on to a wall, countertop, friend, or another stationary object. Do this for five to thirty seconds. Once you've conquered that skill, try standing on one foot without holding on to anything. And then do so while moving your arms in a variety of ways. Playing catch, shaking your booty, and lifting weights while standing on one foot are advanced challenges. And then you can try standing on official balance training tools like the BOSU or balance disks. You can also test your balance by standing on a couch cushion. When standing on squishy objects, start with both feet and eventually move on to single-leg challenges.

The key is to do things that make your feet, ankles, knees, and hips adjust to keep you upright. Done regularly, these exercises will improve your proprioception and decrease your chances of falling.

Circuit Training is a clever way to add variety and save time while exercising. It is done by doing short bits of different exercises without resting in between. This is wise if you'd like to squeeze a quality workout into a condensed period of time. Design your circuit workout by choosing four to 10 different exercises. Commit to doing a predetermined amount of time or reps of each exercise, as well as a certain amount of rounds. Mix and match any sort of exercises to challenge your body and keep yourself entertained. If you alternate between cardiovascular exercises and strength training exercises without resting in between, you'll reap the benefits of an elevated heart rate that come with cardio, even while you're strength training.

Interval Training is done by alternating short bursts of high intensity exercise with longer segments of less intense exercise. It's a fantastic way to increase cardiovascular endurance by adding short bits of intensity into a lengthy workout. If you went to a track, for example, and ran as fast as you could for as long as you could, you might collapse before you completed one lap. Sprinting is anaerobic, which means you're not using oxygen as an energy source. So when you run out of oxygen, you're done! Alternating longer periods of slow running with short bursts of fast running will help increase both your speed and endurance while making your heart and lungs stronger. This model of training can be done with any sort of aerobic exercise. Swim slow for 60 seconds, swim fast for 15 seconds. Cycle slow for two minutes, spin fast for 30 seconds. Choose shorter intense intervals as you start out, and increase them as you become fitter. If you're trying to bounce back from treatment, start with one minute of low intensity and five seconds of higher intensity. Baby steps!

Exercise Instructions

- Mix and match any of these standing, sitting, or horizontal exercises.

- Mix and match bands, dumbbells, and ankle weights, or choose to use no added resistance at all.

- Keep your knees soft when standing, and avoid locking out your knees and elbows throughout each exercise.

- Always work to maintain proper posture.

- Affix bands to stable objects that will not budge when you pull on them.

- Start small when choosing resistance and progress slowly.

- Aim to perform 6-10 repetitions of each strength training exercise. Do less if necessary.

- Aim to hold each stretch for 10-30 seconds.

- Aim to hold balance training exercises for 10-30 seconds

- Don't forget to breathe naturally during each exercise, and avoid holding your breath.

Stretch and Strength Train Anywhere

In this section, you'll learn how to strengthen and stretch each body part. You can do these exercises with any type of exercise equipment, and in any location you choose.

My hopes are that you will commit much of this information to memory, so you will never be able to miss workouts by claiming you didn't know how. I've said it before, but when you know better, you should do better. And when you know how to work each body part, you should be able to train it in the fanciest gym in the world or in the desert. You can also just take this book with you wherever you go!

CHEST

Bench press with Dumbbells

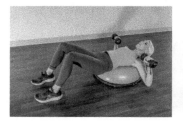 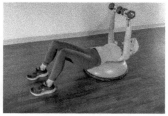

Lie on your back on an elevated surface. Start with your hands near your chest and push forward until your arms are almost straight and your hands are over your shoulders.

Flies with Dumbbells

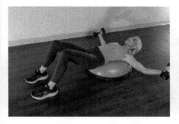
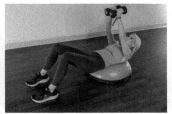

Lie on your back on an elevated surface. Start with your arms almost straight, hands facing each other and over your shoulders. Slowly lower your weights out to the side until your hands line up with your shoulders. Keep elbows soft.

Bench press with Band

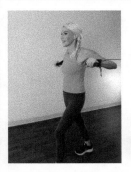
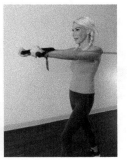

With your bands affixed behind you, stand with soft knees. Start with your hands near your chest and push forward until your arms are almost straight and your hands are in front of your shoulders.

Flies with Band

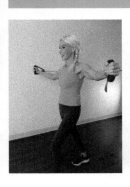
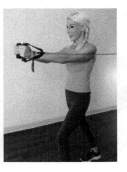

With your bands affixed behind you, stand with soft knees. Start with your arms almost straight, hands facing each other, and chest height in front of you. Slowly bring your arms to the side until your hands line up with your shoulders. Keep elbows soft.

Push-ups

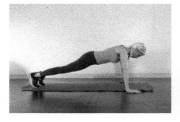
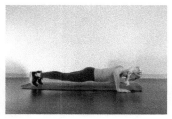

Start in a plank position with hands under your shoulders and a flat back. Lower your body toward the ground and return to starting position.

Flat Back Push-ups on Knees

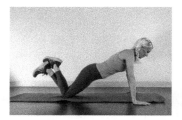
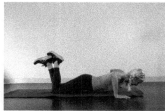

Start on your knees with hands under your shoulders and a flat back. Lower your body toward the ground and return to starting position.

Torso Push-ups on Knees

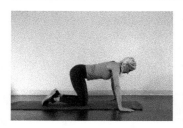
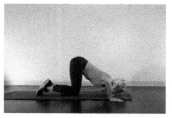

Start with your hips over your knees with hands under your shoulders. Lower your shoulders and chest toward the ground and slowly return to starting position.

Wall Push-ups

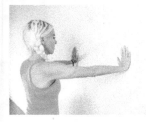

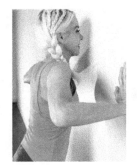

Stand with your hands pressed against a wall at shoulder height with arms only slightly bent. Slowly bring your chest closer to the wall and then push away before you kiss the wall.

Seated Chest and Biceps Stretch

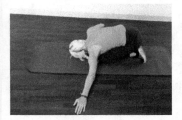

Sit on your knees with your tush resting on your heels. Extend your left arm to one side with your palm on the floor. Press your left shoulder into the floor while rotating your torso to the right.

Standing Chest and Biceps Stretch

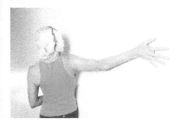

Stand close to a wall with your right arm extended to the side and your right palm pressed against it. Press your right shoulder against the wall and rotate to your left.

BACK

Rows with Dumbbells

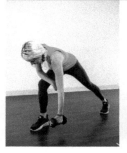 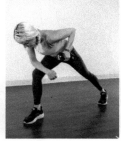

Stand in a lunge position with your left arm resting on your left thigh, flat back. Start with your right arm extended toward the ground. Slowly raise your right hand to your right shoulder.
.

Reverse Flies with Dumbbells

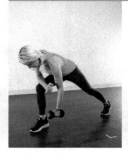 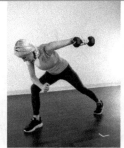

Stand in a lunge position with your left arm resting on your left thigh, flat back. Start with your right arm extended toward the ground and slowly lift it out to the side of your body, ending at shoulder height.

Rows with Band

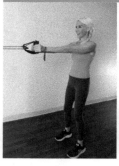 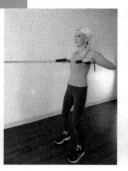

With your band affixed in front of you, stand with soft knees. Start with both arms extended at shoulder height. Slowly pull the band to your shoulders.

Reverse Flies with Band

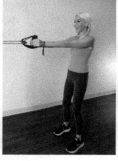 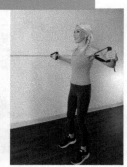

With your band affixed in front of you, stand with soft knees. Start with both arms extended at shoulder height. Slowly pull the band to your sides until they are level with your shoulders. Keep your elbows soft but not fully bent.

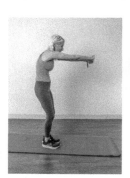

Back Stretch

Stand with soft knees and hands clasped together. Reach your hands far out in front of you while arching your back.

LATS

Lat Pull with Dumbbells

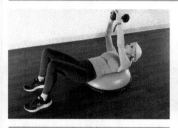

Lie on your back on an elevated surface. Hold one dumbbell with two hands. Start with your arms straight over your chest. Extend your arms behind your head until you can not reach any further.

Lat Pull with Band

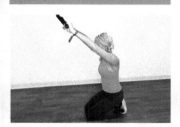

Begin on your knees with your band affixed above you. Holding both handles with your arms extended overhead. Slowly pull your arms toward the ground. Keep your elbows soft but not fully bent throughout the entire motion.

DELTOIDS

Military Press with Dumbbells

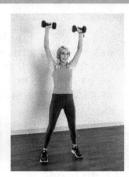

Stand with knees soft and arms up as shown. Press weights toward the ceiling.

Lateral Raise with Dumbbells

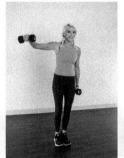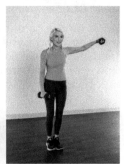

Stand with knees soft and arms extended with hands facing the sides of your thighs. Slowly raise one arm to the side until your hand is level with your shoulder.

Front Raise with Dumbbells

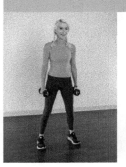

Stand with knees soft and arms extended with hands facing the top of your thighs. Slowly raise one arm in front of you until your hand is level with your shoulder.

Military Press with Band

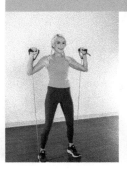

Stand on the center of your band with knees soft and arms up as shown. Extend hands toward the ceiling.

Lateral Raise with Band

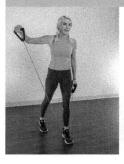

Stand on the center of your band with knees soft and arms extended with hands facing the sides of your thighs. Slowly raise one arm to the side until your hand is level with your shoulder.

Front Raise with Band

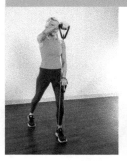

Stand on the center of your band with knees soft and arms extended with hands facing the top of your thighs. Slowly raise one arm in front of you until your hand is level with your shoulder.

Chicken Wing Stretch

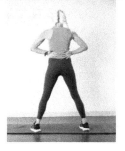

< Place the back of both hands onto your low back and bring both elbows toward the front of your body.

Cross Chest Stretch

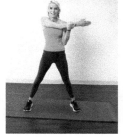

> Bring one extended arm across your chest. Use the opposite hand to pull your extended arm even further across your chest.

BICEPS

Single-arm Biceps Curl with Dumbbells

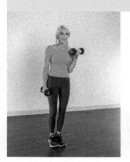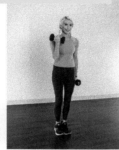

Stand with soft knees with hands at your sides. Keep your elbows pinned tight to your body and slowly bend one arm until your hand is close to your shoulder.

Biceps Curl with Dumbbells

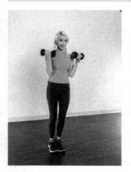

Stand with soft knees with hands at your sides. Keep your elbows pinned tight to your body and slowly bend both arms until your hands are close to your shoulders.

Biceps Curl with Band

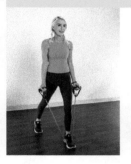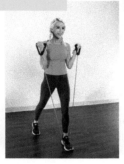

Stand on the center of your band with soft knees and hands at your sides. Keep your elbows pinned tight to your body and slowly bend both arms until your hands are close to your shoulders.

Biceps Stretch

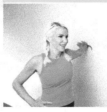

Place one palm against the wall with your fingers pointing behind you. Extend that arm and rotate your body away from the wall.

TRICEPS

Triceps Extension with Dumbbells

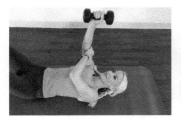 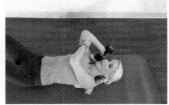

Lie flat on your back with your knees bent. Hold the weight in your right hand with your arm extended straight above your right shoulder. Support your right arm with your left hand to prevent wobbling. Slowly lower the weight toward your right shoulder.

Criss-Cross Triceps Extension with Dumbbells

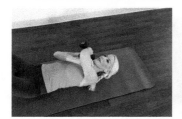 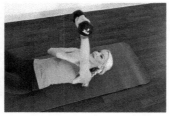

Lie flat on your back with your knees bent. Hold a weight in your right hand with your arm extended straight above your right shoulder. Support your right arm with your left hand to prevent wobbling. Slowly lower the weight toward your left shoulder.

Triceps Extension with Band

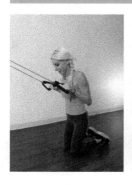 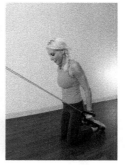

Begin on your knees with your band affixed above you. Holding both handles with your elbows pinned tight at your sides and your hands near your chin, slowly extend your arms toward the ground.

Single-Arm Triceps Extension with Band

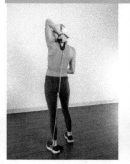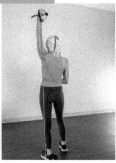

Stand on a band with soft knees. With your left arm bent and your elbow above your head, hold a band handle behind your shoulder. Slowly extend your arm to the ceiling as shown.

Single-Arm Triceps Extension with Dumbbells

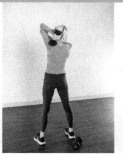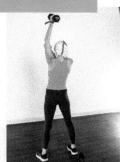

Stand with soft knees. Hold a weight in your left hand with your arm extended straight, reaching up to the sky. Support your left arm with your right hand to keep it stable. Bend your left arm, so the dumbbell drops behind your head. Slowly return to starting position.

Dips on the Floor

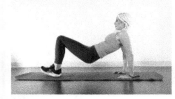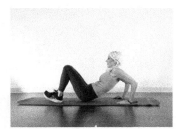

Sit on the ground with your legs in front of you and your knees bent. With hands on the floor behind you and fingers pointed towards your tush, lift your tush off the ground. Slowly bend your arms, lowering your rear to the ground, and then extend your arms to return to starting position.

Triceps Stretch

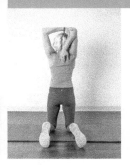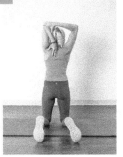

Place your right hand behind your neck with your elbow high. Grab your right elbow with your left hand and gently pull your right arm back. Simultaneously press down on your right forearm with your left thumb to enhance the stretch.

GLUTES & QUADRICEPS

Squat

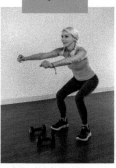

< Sit back until your thighs are parallel to the ground. Do not allow your knees to jet forward over your toes.

Lunge

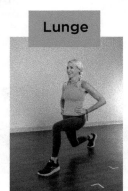

> Take a giant step forward with one leg. Keep your back straight while dropping your back knee toward the ground. Push off of your front foot, bringing your feet back together.

Single Leg Squat

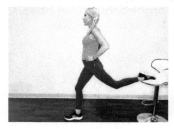

Stand on one foot with your other foot resting on a chair or plyo box. Slowly lower the knee of your back leg towards the ground and return to starting position. Do not allow your front knee to jut forward past your front foot.

Walking Lunges

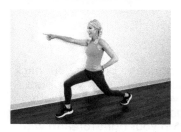

Begin with both feet together. Take a giant step forward with one leg dropping your back knee toward the ground. Bring your back foot up to your front foot. Continue forward, alternating legs

Squat Jump

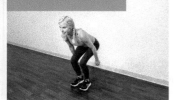

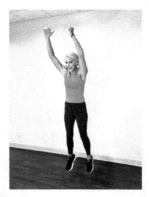

Stand with feet shoulder-width apart. Squat down low and jump up high.

Kick Backs with Band

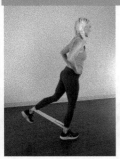

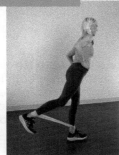

Stand with soft knees and a band looped around your ankles. Keeping toes on both feet pointed forward and knees almost straight, extend one leg backward as far as you can.

Prone Donkey Kicks

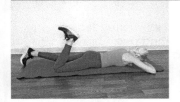

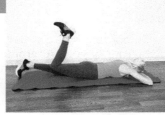

Lie face down with your forehead resting on your hands. Bend one leg and lift your heel to the ceiling. Pulse that foot up and down.

Quad Stretch

Single Leg Folded Glute Stretch

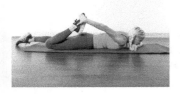

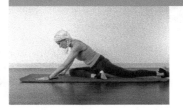

Lay face down on the ground. Grab your right foot with your left hand and bring your foot as close to your tush as possible.

Lean forward over one knee with that foot bent across your body, and extend your other leg behind you.

HIP FLEXORS

Knee Lifts with Band

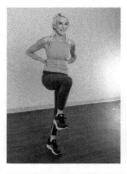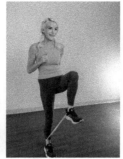

Stand with soft knees and a band looped around your ankles. Keeping toes on both feet pointed forward, alternate lifting your knees as high as possible. Keep your back straight.

Double-Leg V-Up

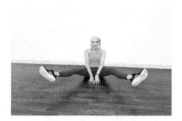

Sit on the ground with both legs in front of you in a "V" shape. Place both hands on the floor between your legs for balance. Simultaneously lift both straight legs off the ground and hold as long as you can.

Single Straight Leg Lifts

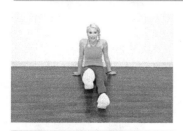

Sit on the ground with both legs extended in front of you. Alternate lifting one straight leg off the ground and holding as long as you can.

Standing Knee Lift

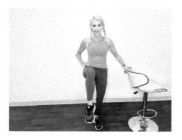

Alternate standing on one foot while holding onto something stable for balance. Lift the opposite knee or straight leg in the air and hold.

Kneeling Hip Flexor Stretch

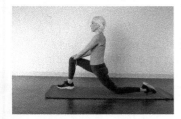

Start in a forward lunge position with your back knee on the ground. Lean your back hip all the way forward.

Kneeling Hip Flexor Stretch Level #2

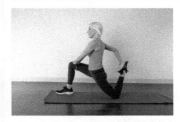

Start in a forward lunge position with your back knee on the ground. Grab your back foot with the opposite hand and lean your back hip forward.

Kneeling Hip Flexor Stretch Level #3

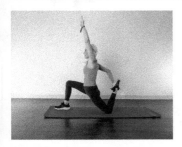

Start in a forward lunge position with your back knee on the ground. Grab your back foot with the opposite hand, reach your other hand to the ceiling and lean your back hip all the way forward.

Standing Hip Flexor Stretch

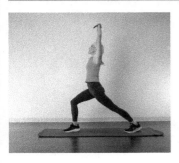

Start in a forward lunge position. Lean your back hip all the way forward. Extend both hands towards the sky.

HAMSTRINGS

Hammy Curls with Band

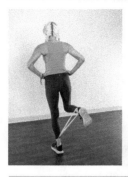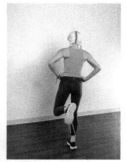

Stand with soft knees and a band looped around your ankles. Keeping toes on both feet pointed forward, alternate bending your legs to kick your tush.

Hammy Stretch

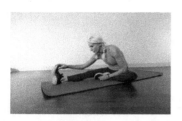

Sit on the floor with one leg extended and one knee bent in a figure-four position. Lower your chest toward your extended leg and hold.

Advanced Hammy Stretch

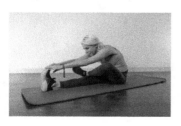

Sit on the floor with one leg extended and one knee bent on top of the extended leg. Lower your chest toward your extended leg and hold.

GLUTE MEDIUS/ABDUCTORS

Lateral Gait with Band

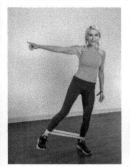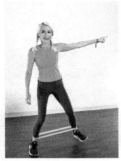

Stand with soft knees and a band looped around your ankles. Take a giant step to the right and bring your left foot in so your feet are together. Take several more giant steps to the right side, and then take several giant steps to your left. Keep your toes pointed forward throughout the exercise.

Lateral Leg Lifts with Band

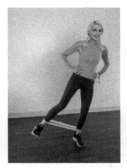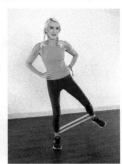

Stand with soft knees and a band looped around your ankles. Keep toes on both feet pointed forward and lift one leg to the side as far as you can. Do several repetitions on that side and then switch legs

Clam Shells

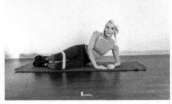

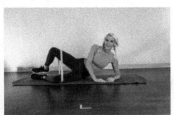

Rest on your side with your knees bent, legs stacked on top of each other, with a band around your thighs, just above your knees. Keeping your feet together, slowly lift your top knee towards the ceiling like you're opening a clam shell.

Lying Lateral Leg Lifts

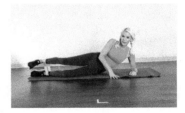

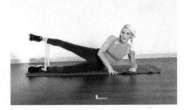

Rest on your side with your legs straight and stacked on top of each other, with a band around your ankles. Keep your legs almost straight with your toes pointed forward, and slowly lift your top leg towards the ceiling.

Criss Cross Applesauce Glute Stretch

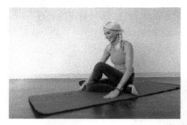 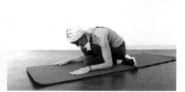

Bend and cross one leg on top of the other. Try to stack your knees on each other (or come close). Lower your chest to your thighs and hold.

ADDUCTORS

Pillow Squeezes

Pillow Squeezes with Bridge

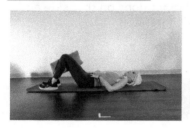 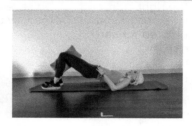

Lay on your back with your knees bent and a pillow or rubber ball between them. Either squeeze your pillow hard for 10-30 seconds or squeeze and release in a pulsing motion.

Lay face up with your shoulders and feet touching the ground and a pillow or rubber ball between your knees. Either squeeze your pillow hard for 10-30 seconds or squeeze and release in a pulsing motion.

Standing Adductor Stretch

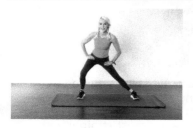

Stand with feet very far apart with toes pointing forward. Bend one knee and shift your weight over to that side.

Army Crawl Stretch

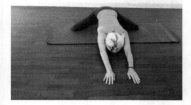
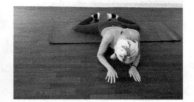

Get on the ground with your knees spread apart, feet together, and your tush seated back on your heels. Lower your hips and chest as much as possible with your arms extended over your head. Keep your hips and chest near the ground and drive your hips forward. Hold both positions for 10-30 seconds.

ABDOMINALS

Plank

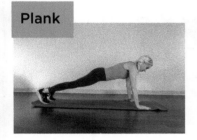

Forearm Plank

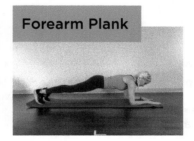

Lie face down on the ground with only your toes and hands touching the floor. Keep your hands directly below your shoulders, and remain still with your body forming a straight line between your heels and shoulders.

Lie face down on the ground with only your toes and forearms touching the floor. Remain still with your body forming a straight line between your heels and shoulders.

Planks with Arm-Lifts

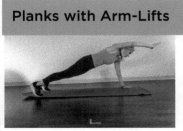
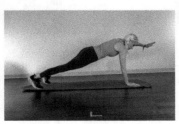

Begin in either plank position and alternate lifting your arms until they're parallel to the ground.

Planks with Leg-Lifts

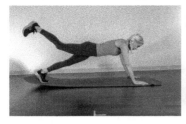 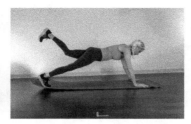

Begin in either plank position and alternate lifting your legs to the ceiling.

Side Plank

Side Plank Leg-Lifts

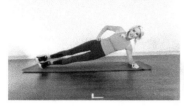 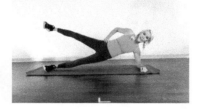

Hold your body up on one elbow (or hand) and the side of one foot. Remain motionless without allowing your lower hip to drop toward the floor.

Begin in the Side Plank position and slowly lift and lower your top leg.

Crunches

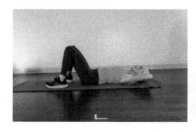 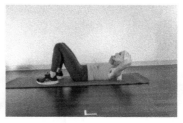

Lie on your back with your knees bent and feet flat on the floor. With your chin high, slowly lift your shoulders off the ground and return to starting position.

Criss-Cross Crunches

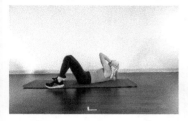 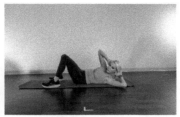

Lie on your back with your knees bent and feet flat on the floor. Keeping your chin high, lift and rotate your right shoulder toward your left knee, then twist and lift your left shoulder toward your right knee.

Straight Leg Criss-Cross Crunches

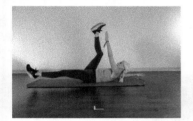 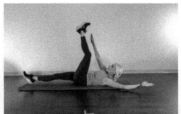

Lie on your back with your legs extended. Keeping your chin high, lift at the shoulder and rotate your right hand toward your left foot. Twist and lift your left hand toward your right foot.

Standing Rainbow Stretch

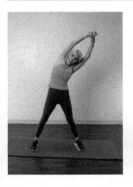 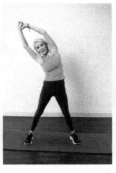

Clasp hands and reach to the ceiling. Lean to one side while reaching high and then the other.

Upward Facing Dog

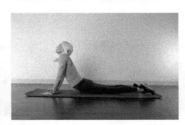

Lie face down with hands below your shoulders. Lift your torso off the ground by extending your arms. Look up towards the ceiling.

ERECTOR SPINAE/LOW BACK

Supermans

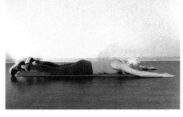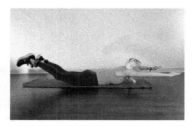

Lie face down with arms and legs extended. Lift both arms and legs off the ground and hold that position for 10-30 seconds.

Swim

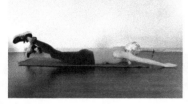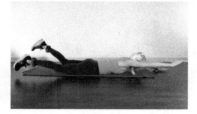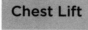

Lie face down with arms and legs extended. Alternate lifting opposing arms and legs as if you are swimming.

Leg Lift

Chest Lift

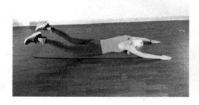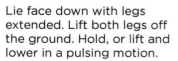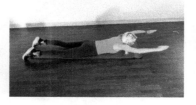

Lie face down with legs extended. Lift both legs off the ground. Hold, or lift and lower in a pulsing motion.

Lift your chest, shoulders, and arms off the ground. Hold, or lift and lower in a pulsing motion.

Bridge

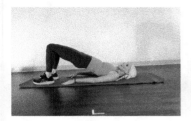

Lay face up with your shoulders and feet touching the ground. Lift your hips so that your body forms a straight line between your knees and shoulders. Hold, or lift and lower in a pulsing motion.

Single-Leg Bridge

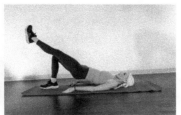

Begin in the basic bridge position and lift one leg so that your body forms a straight line between your foot and your shoulders.

Marching Bridges

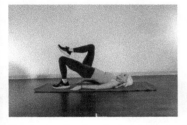
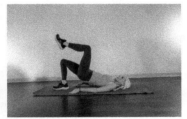

Begin in the basic bridge position and slowly alternate lifting knees in a marching motion.

Angry Cat

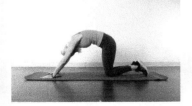

Begin on your hands and knees, and arch your back.

Child's Pose

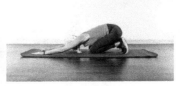

Start on your hands and knees. Sit your tush back on your heels with your arms extended out in front of you.

CALVES

Calf Raises

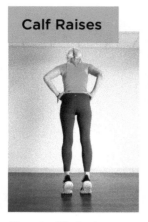

Stand with feet shoulder apart and knees soft. Lift your heels off the ground, rising onto your toes. Hold, or lift and lower in a pulsing motion.

Single-leg Calf Raises

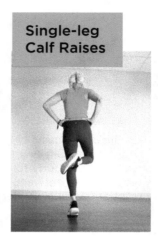

Stand on one foot with your knee soft. Lift your heel off the ground, rising onto your toes. Hold, or lift and lower in a pulsing motion.

Calf Stretch

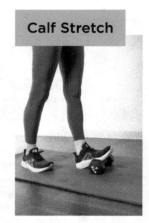

Stand with one foot in front of the other with the forefoot of your front leg elevated onto a dumbbell (or similar height object).

ANTERIOR TIBIALIS

Toe Taps

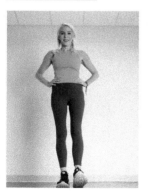

Stand with feet shoulder apart and knees soft. Alternate lifting your toes off the ground.

Weirdo Walk

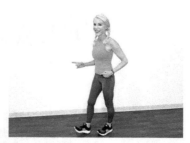

Walk 10-100 steps with your toes lifted, only your heels touching the ground.

Chair Exercises

If exercising standing up doesn't feel good at any point, you can accomplish a whole lot in a seated position or with the support of a chair. You can do these exercises at home, at the office, in a fitness center, and anywhere else. Choose chairs that are comfortable and sturdy, and make movement a priority when doing mundane activities like watching TV. Don't be too shy to do these exercises while sitting in your infusion chair or waiting in exam rooms. Have confidence that you can make tremendous progress with the help of a chair.

Chair fitness classes are growing in popularity at fitness centers everywhere. They cater to a wide variety of people who cannot exercise standing or simply prefer not to do so. They're often really fun and a superb way to socialize. Leave your ego at the door, and get to work!

Flies with Band

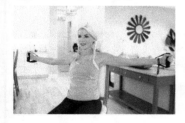 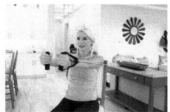

With the band affixed behind you, start with your arms almost straight, hands facing each other, and chest height in front of you. Slowly bring your arms to the side until your hands line up with your shoulders. Return to starting position.

Bench Press with Band

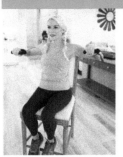 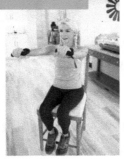

With your bands affixed behind you, start with your hands near your shoulders and push forward until your arms are almost straight at shoulder level.

Military Press with Dumbbells

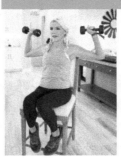 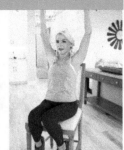

Start with arms wide, elbows bent, and hands facing forward. Press weights toward the ceiling and slowly return to starting position.

Lateral Raise with Dumbbells

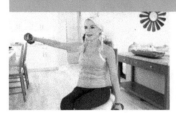 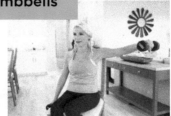

Start with arms extended toward the ground. Alternate each arm to the side until your hand is level with your shoulder.

Straight Leg Lift

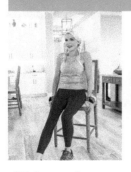 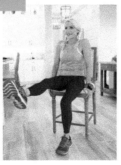

Sit forward on your chair with one leg extended. Slowly lift that leg straight up and down multiple times.

Straight Leg Lateral Lift

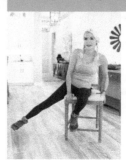 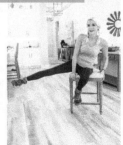

Sit towards the right side of your chair with your right leg extended. Keep your toes pointed forward and slowly lift that straight leg up and down multiple times.

Cardio Flap

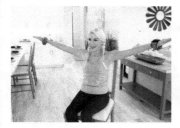
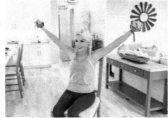

Bring your arms straight out to the side with or without weights and flap your arms up and down like a bird.

Kick Twist

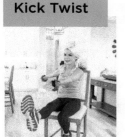
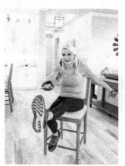

Simultaneously kick one foot while twisting and reaching for it with your opposite hand. Kick, twist, and reach!

March

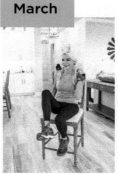
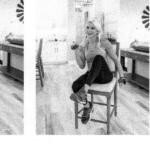

March in your chair by lifting your knees and pumping your arms.

Boxing

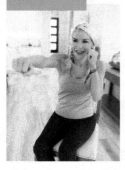
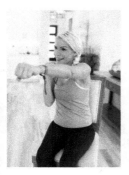

Start with your fists near your face and elbows pinned close to your body. Do a variety of punches on both arms until you've had enough.

Rainbow Stretch

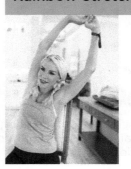
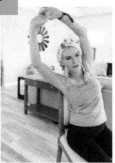

Clasp hands and reach to the ceiling with them. Lean toward each side, making a rainbow with your hands.

Lat Stretch

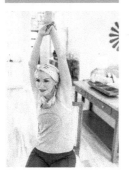

Reach one arm up high overhead. Grab your right wrist with your opposite hand and gently pull your extended arm higher.

Shoulder Stretch

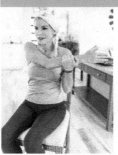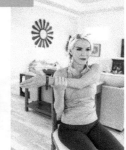

Bring one extended arm across your chest. Use the opposite hand to pull your extended arm even further.

Low Back Stretch

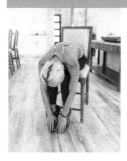

Fold forward in your chair, reaching your hands towards your toes.

Open Chest Stretch

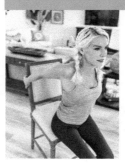

Sit forward on your chair and grab the chair back with both hands. Straighten your arms and lean your chest forward.

Twisty Low Back Stretch

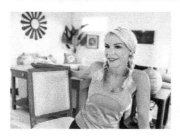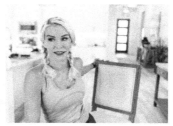

Sit forward in your chair, twist backward, grabbing the left side of your chair back with your right hand. Hold and then switch sides.

Lengthening Stretch

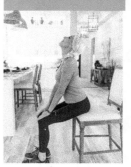

Sit forward on your chair with both feet flat on the floor. Push your chest forward, arch your back and look up.

Angry Cat

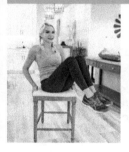

Sit forward on your chair with both feet flat on the floor. Drop your chin and lift your upper back towards the sky.

Hamstring Stretch

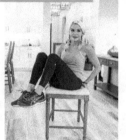

Sit forward in your chair with both legs extended in front of you. Reach towards your toes with both hands.

Piriformis/ Glute Stretch

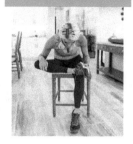

Cross one foot over the opposite knee. Fold your chest forward.

Cardio Lower-Body Twist

Start seated with both feet on the floor, holding onto the sides of your seat. Lift both knees up and to one side. Put both feet back on the floor. Lift both knees in the opposite direction and repeat.

Chair Squats

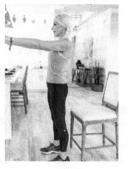
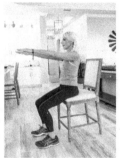

Begin seated normally in your chair. Stand up. Sit back down. Repeat.

Triceps Stretch

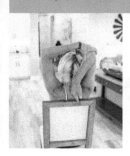
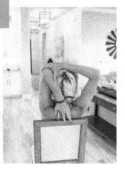

Place your right hand behind your neck with your elbow high. Grab your right elbow with your left hand and gently pull your right arm back. Simultaneously press down on your right forearm with your left thumb to enhance the stretch.

Lateral Leg Lifts

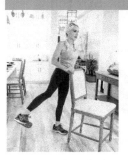

Stand with soft knees using your chair for balance. Keeping all your toes pointed forward, slowly lift one leg to the side and lower it.

Leg Lifts

Stand with soft knees while holding onto your chair for balance. Keeping all your toes pointed forward, slowly lift one leg in front of you and lower it.

Kick Backs

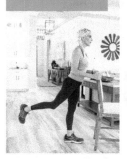

Stand with soft knees while holding onto your chair for balance. Keeping all of your toes pointed forward, slowly lift one leg behind you and lower it.

"No" Neck Stretch

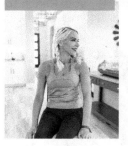

Sit up straight. Keep your chin level (don't look up or down). Slowly look over one shoulder and hold.

Assisted Neck Stretch

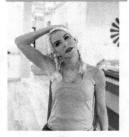

Sit up straight. Keep your chin level (don't look up or down). Place one hand on your head and gently press down, bringing your ear closer to your shoulder.

Abductions with Bands

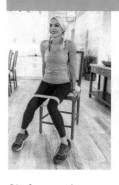
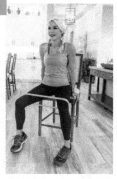

Sit forward on your chair with both feet on the floor and a band wrapped around your thighs (just above your knees). Pull both knees apart and then return to starting position.

Balance with Support

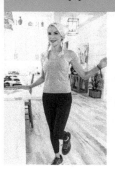

Stand on one foot while holding onto a stable chair, a countertop, a wall, or a friend. If you feel ready for progress, let go of support. Incorporate other balance training exercises near support until you're stable enough to train without it.

Bed Exercises

When cancer and treatments force you into bed, do these exercises when you feel able. Your body will be grateful for the movement.

At home or in a hospital, on the days when you can't walk around or even sit in a chair, these exercises may serve to help you maintain strength, flexibility, and mobility and prevent stiffness. Do them in the mornings, evenings, and during rest periods.

Taller Stretch

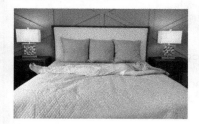

Lie flat on your back with legs straight, and arms extended overhead. Reach in both directions as if you're trying to make yourself taller.

Taller Pillow Stretch

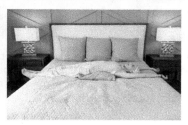

Lie flat with a pillow under your back, legs straight, and arms extended overhead.

Pillow Side Stretch

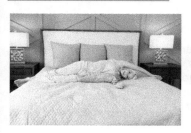

Lie on your side with a pillow under your hips and torso, with legs straight and arms extended overhead.

Prone Pillow Stretch

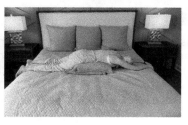

Lie face down with a pillow under your tummy, legs straight, and arms extended overhead. Relax.

Knees to Chest

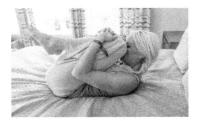

Lie on your back and bring your knees into your chest. Hug your knees tight while tucking your chin into your knees.

Army Crawl Stretch

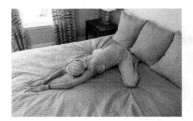 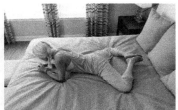

Get on the bed with your knees spread apart, feet together, and your tush seated back on your heels. Lower your hips and chest as much as possible with your arms extended over your head and hold. Keep your hips and chest low and drive your hips forward and hold.

Angry Cat Stretch

Upward Facing Dog

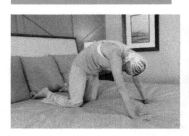 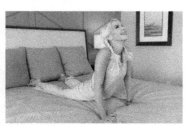

Begin on your hands and knees, and arch your back high.

Lie face down with hands below your shoulders. Lift your torso high off the bed by extending your arms. Look up towards the ceiling.

Quad Stretch

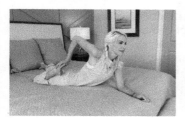

Begin in a prone position with hands below your shoulders. Bend your right leg and grab your right foot with your right hand.

Adductor Stretch

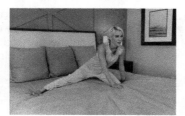

Begin on your left knee with your right leg extended to the side. Shift your upper body weight to your left knee.

Chest and Biceps Stretch

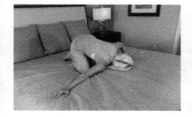 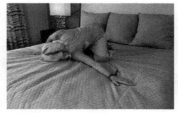

Sit on your knees with your tush resting on your heels. Extend your left arm to one side with your palm on the floor. Press your left shoulder into the bed while rotating your torso in the opposite direction.

Hip Flexor Stretch

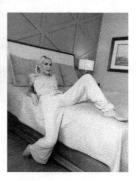

Begin near the edge of your bed with your left leg on the bed and your right leg off the side. Bend your right knee, placing the top of your right foot on the ground.

Low Back Stretch

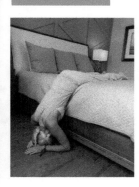

Fold your torso over the edge of the bed, resting your forearms on the ground. Relax.

Side Stretch

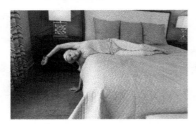

Begin in a side-lying position with your right armpit on the edge of the bed and your right hand on the ground. Reach your left arm up overhead and lean into the stretch.

Extended Twisting Stretch

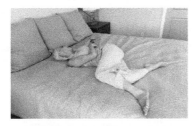

Lie on your back. Cross your left leg over the right side of your body. Twist your torso in the opposite direction looking over the left shoulder.

CrissCross Applesauce Stretch

Headboard Stretch

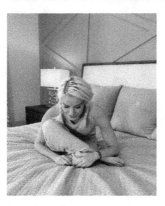

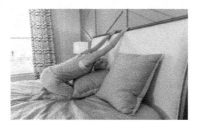

Kneel facing your headboard. Grab the top of your headboard - or the wall near your bed. Sit back on your heels and drop your chest towards the bed.

Bend and cross one leg on top of the other. Try to stack your knees on each other (or come close). Lower your chest and hold.

Hamstring Stretch with Bathrobe Belt

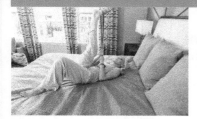

Lie on your back with your left leg bent and your right leg in the air. Wrap the center of your bathrobe belt around your right foot, extend your leg and gently pull the right leg toward your chest.

Adductor Stretch with Bathrobe Belt

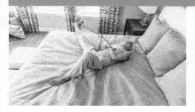

Lie on your back with your left leg bent and your right leg in the air. Wrap the center of your bathrobe belt around your right foot, extend your leg and gently pull the right leg out to the side.

Chest Stretch with Bathrobe Belt

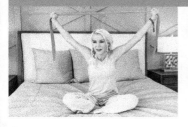
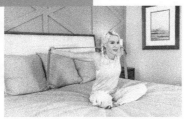

Sit straight up on your bed. Hold a bathrobe belt taut above your head with extended arms. Slowly lower your arms behind you. Loosen your grip on the belt as necessary to complete the motion.

Lateral Leg Lifts

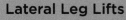
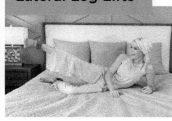

Rest on your side with your legs straight and stacked on top of each other. Keep your top leg almost straight with your toes pointed forward, and slowly lift it towards the ceiling.

Bent-Knee Lateral Leg Lifts

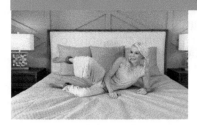

Rest on your side with your legs bent and stacked on each other. Slowly lift it towards the ceiling.

Straight Leg Lifts

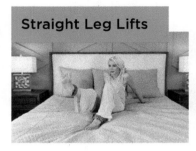 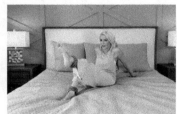

Begin in a reclined seated position with your arms supporting your upper body. Extend one leg in front of you, lifting it up and down.

Crunches

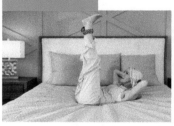

Lie flat with your knees bent or your feet high in the air. Lift your shoulders and lower them.

Lying Triceps Extension

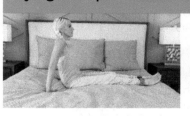 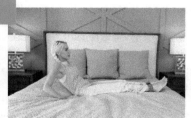

Begin in a seated position with your legs extended. Your straight arms should support your upper body, and your fingers should point toward your tush. Slowly lower your back about 50% of the way toward the bed. Using your triceps and abs, rise back up into starting position.

Bridge

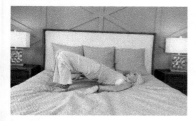

Lay face up with only your shoulders and feet touching the bed. Lift your hips so that your body forms a straight line between your knees and shoulders. Hold, or lift and lower in a pulsing motion.

Marching Bridges

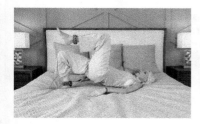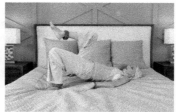

Begin in the basic bridge position and slowly alternate lifting knees in a marching motion.

Single-Leg Bridge

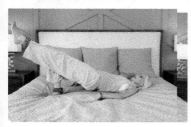

Begin in the basic bridge position and lift one leg so that your body forms a straight line between your extended leg and your shoulders.

Swim

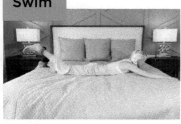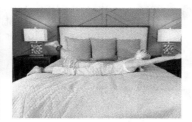

Lie face down with arms and legs extended. Alternate lifting opposing arms and legs as if you are swimming.

Prone Leg Lifts

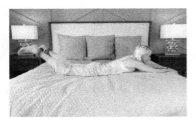

Lie face down with legs extended. Lift both legs off the ground. Hold or lift and lower in a pulsing motion.

Prone Chest Lift

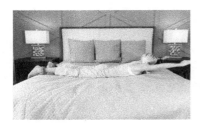

Lie face down with arms and legs extended. Lift your chest, shoulders, and arms off the ground. Hold or lift and lower in a pulsing motion.

Plank

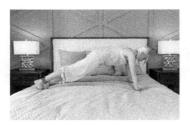

Lie face down on the ground with only your toes, hands, or forearms touching the bed. Keep your hands directly below your shoulders, and remain still with your body forming a straight line between your heels and shoulders.

Side Plank

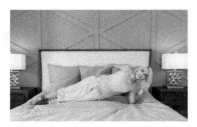

Hold your body up on one elbow (or hand) and the side of one foot. Remain motionless without allowing your lower hip to drop toward the floor.

Upper Body Motions

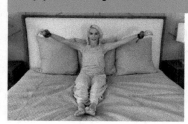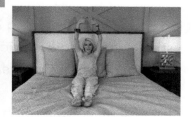

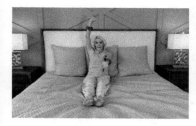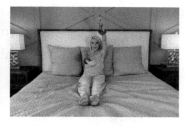

Recline back on some pillows and lift your straight arms up and down in various directions.

Donkey Kicks

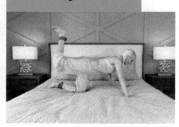

Begin on hands and knees. Lift one bent leg towards the ceiling as if you were trying to kick backward, and return to starting position.

Shower Stretches

Even on super sick days, a little stretching in the shower can feel magical. If you are stable, play some music, move slowly, breathe deeply and enjoy these gentle movements.

The shower is a wonderful place to stretch and relax, but you must show prudence and be cautious not to move quickly or do anything that would result in a fall. Only stretch if the shower floor is a textured non-slip surface, and you feel stable. Safety first!

Soggy Taller Stretch	Soggy Wall Stretch	Soggy Side Stretch

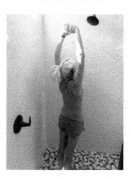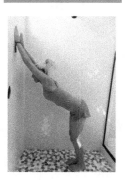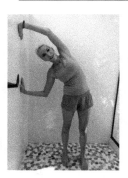

Clasp hands and reach to the ceiling with them	With arms extended, place the palms of your hands against the shower wall and lean forward.	With one side to the wall, place the palms of your hands on the wall - one low and one high. Arch your torso toward the wall.

Soggy Adductor Stretch

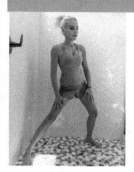

Stand with feet fairly far apart and shift your weight to one side, bending one knee. Stand with feet far apart. Reach up to the sky and over your head.

Soggy Chicken Wing Stretch

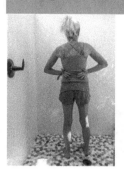

Place the back of both hands onto your low back and bring both elbows toward the front of your body.

Soggy Tricep Stretch

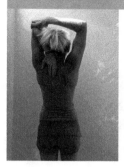

Place your right hand behind your neck with your elbow high. Grab your right elbow with your left hand and gently pull your right arm back. Simultaneously press down on your right forearm with your left thumb to enhance the stretch.

Soggy Angry Cat Stretch

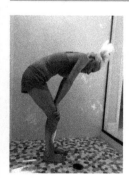

Stand with feet together, and knees slightly bent. Place your hands on your thighs and arch your back toward the sky.

Soggy Standing Chest Stretch

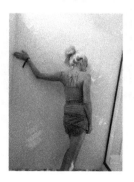

Stand close to a wall with your right arm extended to the side and your right palm pressed against it. Press your right shoulder against the wall and rotate to your left.

Soggy Calf Stretch

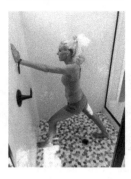

Stand facing a wall in a lunge position with your back leg almost straight, pressing that rear heel to the ground.

Soggy Up and Over Stretch

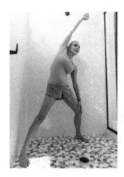

With a wide stance, reach as far up and over as you can.

Soggy Rainbow

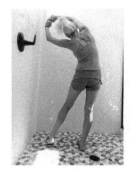

Clench your hands overhead and lean your body from side to side.

Soggy Standing Biceps Stretch

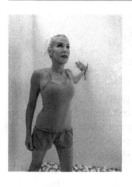

Place one palm against the wall with your fingers pointing behind you. Extend that arm and rotate your body away from the wall.

Soggy Standing Hamstring Stretch

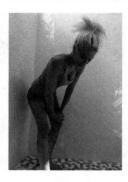

Extend one heel before you, and shift most of your weight onto your base leg. Sit back and lean forward slightly toward the extended leg. Remain mostly upright to avoid tipping over.

Balance Training

Until you're super steady, stand near a wall or another robust and stable object for support. Aim to hold each challenge for 10-30 seconds, but start small, and don't get frustrated if you wobble. Wobbling leads to progress!

Flamingo

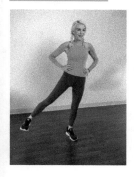

Stand on one foot.

Blind Flamingo

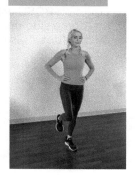

Stand on one foot with your eyes closed.

Flappy Flamingo

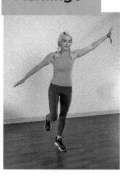

Stand on one foot and move your other leg in various ways.

Kicky Flamingo

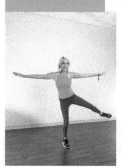

Stand on one foot, reach down and touch the ground.

Flamingo Toe Touch

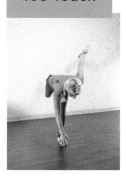

Stand on one foot, reach down and touch the ground.

Firm Flamingo on a Bubble

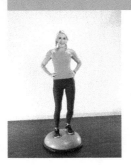

Stand on BOSU with the dome side up on one foot. This is advanced!

Flamingo on a Bubble

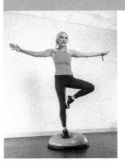

Stand on BOSU with the dome side up on one foot. This is advanced!

CHAPTER EIGHT

Food that Helps vs Food that Hurts

The food you eat shouldn't eat you alive.

Food has the power to help and the power to hurt. In kindergarten, we learned the basics about vitamins, and minerals and how we needed certain amounts of each to help our body function properly. I'm confident it will sound familiar to you when I state that vitamin C can boost your immune system, beta-carotene is good for your eyes, calcium is good for your bones, and protein will help you build muscles. It shouldn't surprise you to learn that excessive sweets, processed foods, and alcohol may do harm. To me, this falls into the category of "common knowledge", but still, many people ignore these lessons learned in our youth and suffer the unpleasant consequences.

Quality nutrition is especially crucial for a cancer patient because treatments may change the way you eat. Digestive troubles may make many foods intolerable and alter the way your body utilizes nutrients. You might need certain foods to boost your energy and build your strength. Additional calories may be required to help you maintain your weight, or fewer calories might be necessary to prevent unhealthy weight gain. Mouth and throat pain might limit you to foods that won't hurt. Perhaps certain pharmaceuticals will place your bone density in harm's way. You should look to nutrition to help you fend off problems while expediting your healing and recovery.

No single food has the proven ability to prevent or cure cancer on its own. But according to the American Institute for Cancer Research (AICR), if your consumption habits include a variety of vegetables, fruits, whole grains, legumes, nuts, and seeds, you can lower your risk for many cancers.[5] On the flip side, there is also convincing evidence to suggest that alcohol (all types - including wine), processed meats (sausages, ham, bacon, hot dogs, salami), and red meats (beef, pork, lamb) increase the risk of certain types of cancer.

Choosing a hot dog over a turkey sandwich in your pre-cancer life might not have seemed like a very big deal, but now it is. Your body needs help and nutritious foods are a powerful way for you to provide it. Sure, your doctors may be serving up a solid can of whoop-ass to your disease. But isn't it better to have multiple cans of whoop-ass when you're fighting an opponent as intimidating as cancer? I think so. And the beauty of choosing nutritious foods as part of your cancer-killing efforts is that there are no negative side effects. No hair loss, burns, or wounds!

As I mentioned in Chapter 1, consulting with a registered dietitian who specializes in oncology is a stellar idea. Your circumstances may require special precautions and your cancer care may be tormenting your digestive system. Just make an appointment and have this important conversation with a professional. Your oncologist should have some recommendations.

Now, let's turn the spotlight on our best and worst food groups. We'll explore some exciting revelations discovered by researchers around the world on nutrition and cancer. Perhaps you'll find that your favorite foods are already working for you. Or maybe you'll take interest in some foods you haven't tried before. Information is KING and once we know better, we tend to do better.

Fruits & Vegetables are packed with vitamins and minerals, and have an extraordinary amount of benefits, especially if you consume a wide variety of each. With regular consumption, they may help lower blood pressure, prevent certain types of cancer, reduce the risks of heart disease, stroke, and Type 2 Diabetes, and aid digestion. They may also have a positive impact on blood sugar levels and help you manage your appetite and body weight.

One of the finest aspects of produce is the convenience factor. You can throw entire oranges, bananas, or apples into your bag in the morning and take them with you for a peel-and-eat experience on the go. Chopped fruits and veggies in containers are perfect snacks for the office, school, or a day outdoors. Tossing frozen produce into a blender with your favorite type of milk or yogurt makes for a delicious and nutritious smoothie. You can also feel confident enjoying produce fresh, frozen, canned, or dried without much change in nutritional benefit. Just steer clear of products with added sugars.

There are thousands of fruits and vegetables with hundreds commonly consumed, so mix it up. Seek out a variety of different tastes, textures, and colors and commit to trying at least one new produce item per week. You may even consider enjoying entire plant-based meals, or committing to a plant-based lifestyle which can provide many benefits. Aim for 7-10 servings per day! Between trying new exercises and eating delicious new foods, your health journey will remain exciting and eye-opening.

Protein is essential to your organs, skin, hair, nails, bones, and virtually every other part of your body. Protein is made up of amino acids which are used to repair muscles and bones as well as create hormones and enzymes. It can also be used as an energy source, as it helps carry oxygen throughout your body in your blood. For practical purposes, you'll recognize that protein is the building block of your muscles, promoting growth and strength. It's also quite filling, so a high-protein meal or snack will render you less likely to overeat or gain weight. Ideal choices include non-fried fish, lean skinless white meats, legumes, nuts, seeds, and eggs. Ask your dietician what your individualized protein goal should be!

Red Meats such as beef, pork, and lamb are fine sources of protein, iron, zinc, and B-12. However, the American Institute for Cancer Research states that there is strong evidence that eating high amounts of red meat increases the risk of colorectal cancer.[6] They recommend eating no more than 12-18 ounces per week if you're unwilling to give it up completely, but less is more. If you do choose to consume red meats, limit them to lean cuts and treat them as a side dish instead of the featured event in your meal. Reduce consumption by substituting lean white meats or soy products in their place, and choosing completely plant-based meals on occasion.

Processed Meats such as bacon, sausage, salami, ham, and hot dogs are classified by the World Health Organization as a Group 1 carcinogen (known to cause cancer). There is strong evidence that processed meats cause cancer, particularly bowel and stomach cancer.[7] Sure they can be convenient and tasty, but the detrimental effects should at least persuade you to cut back dramatically.

Healthy Fats provide energy, support cell function, and help the body absorb important vitamins. There are four different types of fats in food; two are good for you and two you can do without. The good kinds of fats are polyunsaturated and monounsaturated and both decrease your risks for heart disease while lowering your bad cholesterol LDL (low-density lipoprotein). They also boost your good cholesterol HDL (high-density lipoprotein). To help myself memorize which type of cholesterol is good vs bad, I imagine the L in LDL to stand for "lousy" and the H in HDL to represent "healthy", use that trick if you like. Avocados, olives, nuts, and seeds are great examples of healthy fats. Keep in mind that consuming fats does not make you "fat". Fats have a vital role in your body's ability to function, so do not avoid the good kind.

Monounsaturated Fats are liquid at room temperature and harden when chilled. They are good for your brain, skin, and vision and can be found in plant foods such as nuts, avocados, and olive oil.

Polyunsaturated Fats include omega-3 and omega-6 fats which the body needs for brain function and cell growth. We can only get them from food because our bodies do not produce essential fatty acids. They are found in plant and animal foods, including fatty fish (salmon, tuna, mackerel, sardines, and trout) walnuts, soy milk, tofu, sunflower, sesame, and pumpkin seeds.

Trans Fats are formed when vegetables are hydrogenated in an industrial process. This type of fat will harden at room temperature and is often used to keep foods fresh for an extended timeframe. In 2015, the U.S. Food and Drug Administration determined that partially hydrogenated oils (PHOs) are no longer Generally Recognized as Safe in human food, and banned manufacturers from adding them to foods starting in 2018.[8] Their website states that "removing PHOs from processed foods could prevent thousands of heart attacks and deaths each year." You will find trans fats in products like commercial baked goods, shortening, frozen pizza, fried foods, non-dairy coffee creamer, stick margarine, and more. Read labels and if you see the words "hydrogenated oil" or "partially hydrogenated oil," avoid it.

Saturated Fats are mostly found in animal products, with some exceptions, and are typically solid at room temperature. The American Heart Association recommends that they be limited to no more than 6-percent of your daily caloric intake as they can raise your LDL cholesterol.[9] Saturated fats are commonly found in beef, lamb, pork, poultry skin, lard, butter, cheese, ice cream, coconut oil, palm oil, palm kernel oil, and anything baked or fried with these ingredients.

You should avoid artificial trans fats completely if possible, and dial back your consumption of saturated fats. While HDL cholesterol is delivered directly to your liver to be removed from your bloodstream, LDL cholesterol travels straight to your arteries where it can build up potentially leading to heart attacks and strokes.

Whole Grains are naturally high in fiber and filled with nutrients like B vitamins, iron, selenium, magnesium, and potassium. Boosting energy while helping you feel full, they also keep your digestive tract moving and lower your risk of heart disease, certain cancers, and more. Compared to refined and enriched grains, whole grains are consumed in their whole form or ground up into flour while preserving parts of the seed (bran, germ, and endosperm).

You must specifically seek out the term "whole" to ensure you're getting the real deal in products like brown rice, barley, millet, oatmeal, popcorn, crackers, pancakes, and bread. Many products often masquerade as whole grains by using food coloring. Instead of just looking for a brown hue, read nutrition labels in search of the word "whole." The U.S. Dietary Guidelines recommend that Americans make half or all of their grain consumption whole grains. Less than 3-percent of Americans get enough fiber.[10] The American Institute for Cancer Research (AICR) recommends that adults consume at least 30 grams of fiber every day to lower cancer risk.[11]

Legumes are an extraordinary class of vegetables that includes beans, peas, lentils, and peanuts which are packed with a surprising amount of nutrients. Nutrition varies by type, but you can often expect protein, calcium, folate, iron, fiber, magnesium, and antioxidants. According to the National Library of Medicine, regular consumption can lower your risk of certain types of cancers, Type 2 Diabetes, and heart disease.[12,13] They can also benefit your digestive system including the gut microbiome, muscles, and more. Legumes are an ideal protein choice for a plant-based lifestyle since they offer many of the nutrients one would seek out in meat.

Legumes are usually easy to access and affordable. You can get them in bags, cans, in the frozen-food section, or at your farmer's market. They're also commonly enjoyed in dips, spreads, soups, and chilis. Try chickpeas, peanuts, lentils, hummus, and beans and peas of all sorts.

Nuts and Seeds pack so much quality into a tiny little space. The nutrition in each varies by type, but you can find protein, calcium, good fats, omega-3 and omega-6 fatty acids, antioxidants, and more. Regular consumption can benefit brain function, skin and hair growth, bones, the reproductive system, metabolism, and digestion. It can also lower your risk of certain cancers, heart disease, and inflammation-induced issues. Many associate nuts with weight gain, but that's true only if you overdo it. They are dense with calories, but consuming a few ounces of a variety of nuts per day can have enormous benefits, making them anything but "empty calories". Because they require no refrigeration, they are convenient and their shelf-life is quite long. Choose nut butters without added oil, and nut-based milks. Include seeds and nuts in recipes or make your own custom bags of trail mix.

All-Mighty Water

Approximately sixty percent of the human body is comprised of water, and those water levels require constant refreshing. Water is vital to breathing, heart health, digestion, liver, kidney, and brain function, muscular mobility, and more. Being dehydrated means more than just being thirsty. It means that your body parts and systems are being deprived of one of their essential requirements to function properly. Think about what happens to your favorite plant when you forget to water it. Unless it's one of those unique desert varieties, plants go limp pretty quickly without sufficient water. So do we! You may not even realize that your headache, dizziness, crankiness, forgetfulness, hunger, muscle soreness, or nausea is a result of dehydration. With all the hardships you're already enduring, preventing added misery due to dehydration is a pretty easy fix. Make a habit of keeping a large bottle of water with you and sip from it regularly.

Not only will your body work less efficiently without proper hydration, but the effects of dehydration feel really bad! When my dehydration became extreme, my doctor brought me in for daily IV fluids which were very helpful. Perhaps this might be a solution for you as well. At the beginning of my treatment, a friend who'd fought her cancer battle years prior gave me some golden advice. She said "I know you're getting all sorts of unsolicited and unwanted advice from everyone. The only pointer I'm going to share is to drink lots of water." I thought of her words often, drank more than I would have because of them, and I do believe my deliberate effort helped. How could it not?

Chemotherapy, radiation, and many pharmaceuticals can be dehydrating, so you must fight back. Water is the gold standard for hydration, but many other beverages will do the trick. Electrolyte beverages may even be required on occasion, but avoid added sugar. Fruits and veggies can also be quite hydrating, which is another reason to choose them at snack and mealtime as often as possible.

Percentage of human body parts comprised of water:

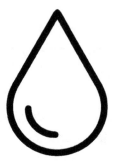

- Brain 73%
- Heart 73%
- Skin 64%
- Pancreas 73%
- Liver 71%
- Muscles 79%
- Kidney 79%
- Lungs 83%
- Bones 32%
  According to H.H. Mitchell, *Journal of Biological Chemistry* 158[14]

Processed Foods are any raw agricultural product that has been altered in any way from its original form. Processing isn't always bad as long as the changes are minimal and they do not lessen the nutritional value of the raw food product. Minimally processed foods include chopped vegetables, roasted nuts, or dehydrated fruit. This level of processing preserves nutrition without creating any downsides. However, processing should make you leery when preservatives, hydrogenated oils, excessive sugar and salt, and other problematic ingredients are added. These additives can turn a nutritious raw food item into an unhealthy choice in a hurry. It's actually quite sad when quality food is completely bastardized. Frozen peaches, for example, are a fantastic choice because they were quickly peeled and frozen soon after being picked, maintaining most of their nutrition. Canned peaches in sugary syrup, on the other hand, are far less wonderful. Potatoes are bursting with vitamin C and potassium, and are a quality source of carbohydrates. They may do more harm than good once they become French fries or chips. Ready-to-eat snacks and meals such as crackers, deli meats, and frozen dinners are often packed with preservatives and high levels of sodium. Besides being a culprit for weight gain and obesity, a study published in *The British Medical Journal* found that ultra-processed foods are linked to an increased risk for cancer, so read labels and avoid them as much as possible.[15]

Limit these processed foods:
- Sugary soft drinks
- Shelf-stable meals
- Packaged baked goods and breads
- Instant noodles and soups
- Sweet or savory packaged snacks
- Processed meats such as deli meats, bacon, hot dogs, chicken nuggets, fish sticks, chorizo, ham, pastrami, pepperoni, and salami.
- Any food products made mostly or entirely from sugars, oils, and fats

Choose foods and ingredients in their most natural form, or as close to it as possible. Read labels and if the ingredients aren't easily identifiable to you as something that once grew from the ground, or if you can't pronounce them, you might want to make another choice.

Alcohol is a World Health Organization class I carcinogen. Liquor, beer, wine, etc. According to the U.S. Center for Disease Control, the less alcohol you drink, the lower your risk for cancer.[16] Alcohol increases your risk for many forms of cancer. Mouth and throat, voice box (larynx), esophagus, colon and rectum, liver, and breast (in women). The reason alcohol increases your risk for cancer is that it actually can damage your DNA. DNA controls normal cell growth and function. But when DNA is damaged, a cell can begin growing out of control and create a cancerous tumor.

For many, alcohol is a source of fun, socialization, relaxation, and stress management. However, the consequences are often grave. Accidents, injuries, addiction-induced hardships, legal ramifications, monetary losses, confrontations, and illness. The fact that consumption may also lead to cancer should be sufficient motivation for you to stop completely or reduce the role of alcohol in your life. Yes, this includes wine. All wine.

Sugar consumption is often connected to cancer growth, but studies haven't yet proven a direct link. However, there is an indirect link that should be taken seriously. High consumption of sugary beverages, including fruit juice, snacks, and food products, may lead to weight gain and excess body fat. The Dana-Farber Cancer Institute states that research shows that being overweight or obese increases the risk of 11 types of cancers, including colorectal, postmenopausal breast, ovarian, and pancreatic cancer.[17]

Refined sugar consumption has also been associated with Type 2 Diabetes, acne, tooth decay, expedited aging, depression, fatty liver disease, and more. Can you live without sugar? Yes! Do you have to cut sugar out completely?

Not necessarily. Instead, reserve sugary sweets for rare occasions. Dump sugary beverages from your daily habits, doughnuts from your breakfast menu, and candy from your lunchbox. If you feel good about celebrating your birthday or a team victory with cake or a trip to an ice cream parlor, go for it!

Supplements. It's terrifying how many people self-prescribe supplements or take "nutrition" advice from random friends or minimum-wage salespeople at "nutrition stores" who have absolutely no legitimate expertise. For the average person, this practice often wastes a ton of money and creates potential health risks. For cancer patients and survivors, the outcomes can be much worse. It's not to say that supplements can't play a productive role in your health, but it's vital to choose only those that will help without doing harm. Radiology oncologist Dr. Allison Grow says, "Many people feel that they need various supplements to optimize their diet to beat cancer (partly because of aggressive manufacturer marketing). High-quality evidence is almost always lacking, and some supplements actually potentiate toxicities of treatment (e.g. many Chinese herbal preparations have blood thinning properties, many high-dose vitamin therapies can be nephrotoxic or accumulate to toxic levels in fat cells, etc). For the macro- and micronutrients your body needs, look to whole foods to optimize your eating habits rather than piling on the supplements. I'm definitely not opposed to all supplements, I take some myself, but megadoses (more than 5X the US RDA) should generally be avoided, and there should be full mutual disclosure between patients, doctors, and all complementary therapists." [18]

Overall, aim to eat a wide variety of fresh whole foods in their natural form and avoid processed foods as much as possible. Most foods grown from the ground are excellent nutrition sources with plentiful benefits. The more steps a food item has endured before arriving on your plate, the less nutritious it will likely be. As well, keep your water bottle filled and nearby, and constantly work on drinking it. A well-nourished and well-hydrated body can do extraordinary things.

Keep track of your progress, set goals, and record memories with the *Healthy Cancer Comeback Journal*!

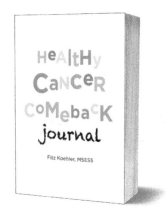

CHAPTER NINE

Not too Big, Not too small... Just Right

Even though weight loss, weight gain, and weight management are often made out to be the most confusing things in the world, the formula for it all is actually quite simple. Cancer care is often thought to be associated with dramatic weight loss, but the reality is that a much greater percentage of breast cancer patients, for example, gain weight during treatment. Breast Cancer Lifestyle Medicine Specialist Dr. Dawn Mussallem advises that instead of creating a weight-loss plan during treatment, patients should focus on "not gaining weight." She says that studies have shown only 10-percent of patients will be able to lose the weight they gained during treatment, and this added weight will diminish long-term prognosis.[19] It's a tough situation, but it's important that you do your best to maintain a healthy weight. You and your doctor should discuss exactly what that weight is. I promise that if you follow the Exact Formula you will be able to lose, gain or maintain your weight exactly how you'd like to if outside influences like steroids do not interfere.

I'm going to share a bunch of basic science and math with you here, but I want you to receive it without stress or pressure. This is a time to show true compassion for yourself, and quite often weight management yields the opposite. Instead of thinking "I'm too fat" or "I'm too skinny," eat with absolutely nothing but health and quality of life in mind. Your weight can and will definitively affect your health, so this is a wonderful way to take control. Chapter 1 was brimming with talk about control, so I hope you'll proceed with the topic of weight management knowing that the closer you are to your ideal weight, the better your chances are for longevity. Never beat yourself up. This isn't the time to agonize over your appearance. Instead, focus on your ideal or "fighting weight" and all of the benefits that come with it.

Beyond basic math, the Exact Formula requires a deep appreciation for the fact that your body needs calories to function. It's also important to know that when it comes to weight management, your body will do what you tell it to. I liken it to setting the thermostat in your home. Just because you've set the temperature to become 72-degrees doesn't mean your house will immediately change. Instead, you point your thermostat to a certain temperature and with time and effort by your air conditioner or heater, your temperature goals are met. Achieving your ideal weight is the same. You constantly have to direct your body to your desired weight and eventually, it will get there.

On average, humans burn about 10 calories per day per pound of body weight. If you weigh 200 pounds, your body will likely burn about 2,000 calories each day just to maintain its size and normal body function. That's not counting exercise. It's just the amount of calories your body will burn doing important things like digesting food, pumping blood, processing oxygen, walking around the house, brushing hair—standard stuff. Every move we make requires energy, thus calories get burned. If you burn about 2,000 calories a day and you are maintaining your weight, we know that you're also consuming at least 2,000 calories a day.

2,000 calories in vs 2,000 calories burned = no change
3,500 extra calories consumed = one pound gained
3,500 extra calories burned = one pound lost

If you presently weigh 200 pounds but have a healthy or preferred weight of 150 pounds, you'll need to lose 50 pounds. Our simple math says that if you'd like to weigh 150 pounds, you should eat the proper amount of calories that would sustain a person no bigger than 150 pounds. 150 x 10 calories per day = 1,500. At 200 pounds, you're consuming at least 2,000 calories per day, and that's too much! That's the reason you're 50 pounds overweight. You've been eating to be a 200-pound person.

The beauty of the formula is that it works in both directions and is incredibly simple. If you are trying to gain weight, you simply must consume the number of calories required to weigh that much. If you weigh 140 pounds but prefer to weigh 200 pounds, you're going to have to eat far more than you have been to pack on 60 extra pounds, at least 2,000 calories a day. It will not likely happen overnight and you may not find eating so much to be as "fun" as most people make weight gain out to be. But you might. And I hope you do.

Lastly, if you've been coasting at your ideal weight for a while and are hoping to not gain or lose anything during or after cancer care, do the math and continue to stick with your caloric budget. If you weigh 175 pounds and you love it, set a target of 1,750 calories daily and you shouldn't see much of a difference.

How do you customize this formula for you? Easy! Decide what a healthy weight for you would be, and then tack a ZERO onto the end of it. That provides you with 10 calories per pound of ideal body weight, and by sticking to this caloric budget, your body will move toward your ideal weight. You will be feeding it enough to function well at your ideal weight while denying it the ability to remain at a size you do not prefer.

Caloric Budgets for Weight Loss

Want to weigh 214 pounds? Consume no more than 2,140 calories per day

Want to weigh 132 pounds? Consume no more than 1,320 calories per day.

Caloric Budgets for Weight Gain

Want to weigh 214 pounds? Consume at least 2,140 calories per day

Want to weigh 132 pounds? Consume at least 1,320 calories per day.

Caloric Budgets for Weight Maintenance

Want to continue weighing 214 pounds? Consume 2,140 calories per day.

Want to weigh 132 pounds? Consume 1,320 calories per day.

This formula works EVERY TIME! It's NOT a diet, it's just a method of managing your consumption habits (both food and beverage) to ensure you're providing your body with the ideal amount of energy (calories) and not an excessive amount.

You can do this the smart way or the dumb-dumb way. The dumb-dumb way would have you eat low-quality high-calorie foods like doughnuts each day and nothing else. YES, you can consume 1,500-2,000 calories with just a few doughnuts and still lose or gain weight. However, with this methodology, you'd have no energy, be tired, malnourished, hungry, have headaches, grow cranky and quit. This dumb-dumb plan is not built for success.

The SMART way to attack this formula is by filling your daily caloric budget with tons of HIGHLY NUTRITIOUS foods. If you want to have energy and feel satisfied while enjoying what you eat, choose unprocessed high-fiber items including vegetables, fruit, whole grains, legumes, nuts, and seeds. When selecting animal sources be sure to select lean proteins. Avoid sugary high-calorie beverages including fruit juice, processed foods, alcohol, and saturated and trans fats as much as possible. Yes, I'm suggesting that you have really high standards most of the time. Perfection is almost impossible to attain, so if you'd like to set aside 10%-15% of your daily intake for "fun calories" go ahead and do so.

Remember, you are NOT on a diet. Diets are temporary, drastic measures that yield short-term results and long-lasting aggravation. Instead, you are just going to start becoming particular about what and how much you are putting in your mouth. Fill up on the great stuff and scrutinize the high-calorie non-essentials. Could you broil that chicken breast instead of frying it? Sure you can! Can you dip your salad in a side cup of dressing instead of allowing the restaurant to dump ladles on top of it or better yet just squeeze lemon juice or pour a little balsamic vinegar on top? You betcha! Can you choose another way to relax each night instead of having that glass of wine or beer? Unless you've got an addiction, you can and if you have an addiction ask yourself if you are ready for help.

Folks, weight management shouldn't feel like torture. If it does, then what you're doing isn't sustainable. Weight management can and should be simple: learn what works for your body, stay within reasonable parameters and make more good choices than bad.

FAQ's

When I lose weight, can I go back to eating more calories?
No. If you want to be a smaller person permanently, you'll have to continue to eat like a smaller person. You may find a place where you can eat a bit more based on a vigorous exercise routine, but if you veer too far from your formula,. you'll eventually gain weight.

Can I splurge?

It's YOUR caloric budget and you don't have to be perfect. Perfect is boring! Just make great choices and stick to your budget 90-percent of the time. I eat a small piece of milk chocolate which I know is inferior to dark chocolate every single day. It makes me happy.

If I exercise, do I eat more to compensate for the calories burned?

Not if you're trying to lose weight. Purposely re-consuming calories you just burned to lose weight would be insane! That would be like quickly spending the $1,000 you just earned on a fancy purse when you were trying to save up to buy a $15,000 car. Unless you are doing over an hour of vigorous exercise, you likely do not need to purposely re-consume the calories you've burned off. Many apps and "diets" tell you to do this, and all I can say is ... FOOEY! They're unknowledgeable amateurs who have no business guiding you toward weight loss. If you burn an extra 500 calories per day through exercise, you will lose an extra pound a week. If you burn 500 calories and quickly re-consume them, you will lose zero extra pounds each week.

Now, if you are trying to gain or maintain your weight, then yes. You may consume more to make up for the difference.

My husband gets to eat way more than I do. Is it fair? Maybe not, but you'll probably prefer being fit and lean over keeping up with his luxurious eating abilities. If you eat like a big man, you will weigh the same.

How do I keep track of calories? Great question! I recommend a free app like My Fitness Pal. Just plug in every bite and sip you take each day and when the app says you've reached your limit ... stop eating. If you're trying to gain weight, don't stop consuming until you've reached your goal. You can also jot down notes with a pen and paper to keep track if you're not tech-savvy.

Should I add exercise? Of course! You can be trim without exercise, but you cannot be FIT without it. We talked about this in Chapter 3. Exercise is a powerful force in weight management, but more importantly, exercise is the only way to become strong and flexible, with good balance and endurance. Skinny is no prize! Your goal should be lean and strong.

What if I hate counting? Too bad. Plug the numbers into your phone, computer, or *Healthy Cancer Comeback Journal* and enjoy the benefits. I bet you dislike being overweight or underweight more than you dislike counting. Do you keep track of the money you spend to ensure you don't accidentally drain your account or bounce checks? I bet you do. Counting and simple math are a part of being a responsible adult. Keeping track of your healthy habits like this will also help you hold yourself accountable and celebrate your progress along the way.

What if I hate scales? That's like saying you hate thermometers or rulers. Scales are simply tools of measurement. They don't love you, hate you, or care if it's the holiday season. They just tell you the truth and let you make decisions based on that information. Your weight is not the only important factor, but you're learning about the formula because you care about your weight. Don't bury your head in the sand. Check in with a scale regularly; I recommend weekly. If the scale is moving in the right direction, you know you've been doing a good job. If the number is sticking or going the wrong way, you'll know to tighten up a bit and put in a little more effort.

I'm trying to gain weight, so can I consume more calories than my formula suggests? Absolutely! For the general population, I recommend both gradual weight loss and gradual weight gain. However, if cancer has wreaked havoc on you and you're just way too thin, go ahead and pile on the calories if you can. As with anything, I recommend choosing high-quality nutrition. Good foods will do great things for your body and right now, your body needs all of the support it can get. Fruits, vegetables, nuts, and beans are brimming with immune-boosting nutrients that can help you fight your disease. Do you need to be perfect with nutrition? Not necessarily. Just choose wisely as often as possible. Baked French fries taste just as yummy as fried French fries. Make the extra effort when you can.

What about the 1,200 calorie-a-day message I've always heard? It's preposterous to think that a random amount of calories would suit everyone. A large football player would STARVE if that's all he was fed each day. 1,200 calories is a completely random number that does not take into account various heights, weights, body types, or goals. With the Exact Formula, you get to choose your goal weight based on those factors. Your formula is created specifically for you. Reaching fitness goals, especially during cancer treatment, looks completely different for everyone.

What if I feel hungry all of the time? Increase your intake of protein, healthy fats, and fiber. This will increase your feelings of satiety or fullness.

Do I have to count calories forever? I do. I don't plug them into an app anymore, but I do keep mental notes throughout the day. Sidebar - I used to weigh 45 pounds more than I do now. I wore sizes 13-15 back then and wear a 2 now. I taught two intense group fitness classes a day back when I was overweight too. What changed? My eating habits. And, when chemo caused me to lose about 10% of my weight, I used the Formula to gain it back in a healthy way. Other than during my time as a cancer patient and during pregnancies, I've maintained a weight I love for over 20 years, just by being a conscientious eater. So many people around the globe have already used and found success using the Exact Formula. Those who achieve and maintain their ideal weights are those who stick to the formula no matter what.

What do I do when I achieve my goal weight? Plan a fun athletic adventure to celebrate, buy a few new outfit you feel fantastic in and commit to the Formula for the rest of your life. Why would you ever stop doing something that brought you success?

What is my ideal weight? There are tons of charts and graphs that I could share here, but I won't. Far too often, I see the BMI calculator tell muscular athletes and curvy fit women they are overweight. I have great confidence that between you and your doctor, you can pick a weight to aim for with good health in mind. As you close in on your original goal weight, you can make rational adjustments. I believe most people know their fighting weight.

CHAPTER TEN

Complementary care & other stuff to make you feel good

In addition to your efforts with exercise, nutrition, sleep, and mental fitness, there are a variety of complementary care options you can pursue to relax, recover, heal, and grow stronger. The big "C" can hit a person at all sorts of angles, so it's equally wise to use every offensive and defensive tool you can to keep the bad stuff at bay. Chat with your medical team before you add anything new to make sure nothing will be more harmful than helpful. Ask for recommendations whenever possible and remember that some of these services might be covered by insurance if you have it. You may want to request prescriptions.

Acupuncture

This ancient form of Chinese medicine is said to stimulate the body's natural healing processes to relieve or resolve all sorts of dreadful issues. For cancer patients, it's commonly used to reduce neuropathy, decrease nausea, increase energy and reduce anxiety. While needles are usually involved, they are incredibly thin and far gentler than those used for chemo and blood draws. Even needle-phobes (like me) can get comfortable with the practice and enjoy its benefits.

Mental Health Counseling

Cancer can cause inordinate amounts of stress which can affect your physical, emotional, and social well-being. This stress can disrupt your sleep, eating habits, relationships, ability to work, and more. Suffering silently won't win you any prizes, and seeking help doesn't mean that you are mentally ill. Talking to a professional may help you cope, achieve calm, find perspective, and muster strength. Research has shown decreased adherence to treatment plans and poorer health outcomes for cancer patients struggling with mental health. It can be difficult to have honest conversations with loved ones, so this option may be the perfect way to alleviate your stress and move forward positively.

Support Groups

Discussing your situation with others fighting cancer can be incredibly comforting. They say, "misery enjoys company", but I think it's more appropriate to say that company diminishes misery. I found it much easier to laugh at myself and the insanity of my experiences when talking with friends who were also going through it. Attending a support group might serve as the perfect place for you to have honest and guilt-free conversations with strangers who care. Besides providing comfort and encouragement for each other, you may pick up some brilliant tips for dealing with random side effects that only someone in a similar predicament could know. Your medical team and local cancer nonprofit may be able to refer you to an appropriate group.

Online support groups are incredibly popular now and could be a fantastic alternative if you don't prefer to connect in person. I recommend seeking out groups that are professionally monitored. Without it, conversations might become more negative than encouraging. You also don't want to end up in a group with evil-doers lurking and working to take advantage of you.

Massage Therapy

Besides having the potential to feel fabulous, having a licensed massage therapist rub and manipulate your body's soft tissues (muscle, connective tissue, tendons, ligaments, and skin) can serve a ton of wonderful purposes. Quality massages can remove pain, increase range of motion, break up scar tissue, alleviate neuropathy and induce relaxation. A therapist can utilize a variety of techniques under or over your clothes to promote healing and help you recover. If you're dealing with lymphedema, an experienced professional may be able to help. Manual Lymphatic Drainage Massage involves techniques designed to help reduce the build-up of fluid.

Physical Therapy

Think of a physical therapist as a medically-superior version of a personal trainer. Expect a physical therapist to evaluate your strengths, weaknesses, and limitations, and design a personalized and comprehensive game plan for rehabilitation. Their efforts may include strengthening and stretching exercises, massage therapy, dry needling, electric stimulation, ultrasound, heat, ice, and more. You may see a physical therapist in the hospital, in a physical therapy facility, or your home. If you are facing any physical limitations, this is an ideal place to start.

Sexual Health Counseling

Often ignored, this can be a struggle for many going through treatment and their partners. Sickness, fatigue, vaginal dryness, erectile dysfunction, physical changes, pain, scars, depression, and more. Specifically addressing sexual organs, it's not surprising that a woman might feel uncomfortable with her body after having a full or partial mastectomy. Men might agonize over having testicles removed. Changes to our bodies such as scars, amputations, ports, ostomies, and more could diminish body confidence, libido, and performance. Intimacy may also be disrupted, even if only because a loving partner is concerned about hurting the patient. A healthy relationship with your body and your partner (if you have one) can be healing and comforting, both physically and emotionally. A healthy sex life may also serve to improve self-esteem, enhance sleep, decrease depression, lower blood pressure and bring joy.

Orgasms release the pleasure hormone oxytocin into your body causing all sorts of good things to happen. So even if you don't have a romantic partner, plan on having some orgasms by yourself. Most of the benefits remain and you can just chalk it all up to healthiness! Talk to your doctor and ask for a referral to a specialist. Don't be shy! Your doctor has heard everything before and will likely help if given the opportunity.

Meditation

Meditation is the practice of using focus and mindfulness to calm the mind and manage emotions. Evidence shows that this self-soothing effort can relieve depression, anxiety, and pain while improving sleep and lowering blood pressure. You can meditate in any quiet place where you will focus on words, physical actions, objects, or breathing. If you'd like instruction, download an app or seek guidance online. Meditation does not require an appointment and can be done alone and without cost. It has zero downsides and if you practice regularly, it may make a positive impact on your health.

Hair & Nail Growth Products

Boy, do I wish I had some sort of practical and effective guidance here. Trust me. I've researched every cream, lotion, shampoo, and supplement on earth looking for a quick fix, or even a slow fix, with no success. Like many of you, during my lengthy period of head-to-toe baldness, my desire to grow some hair back was intense. I also wanted a solution for my fingernails and toenails which turned yellow, bumpy, stinky, and rotted out. Eventually, they all ripped off, which was both painful and frustrating. Sadly, a realistic solution for my situation did not exist. I only tell you this because I understand the desperation and I don't want you to be bullied, suckered, or tricked into spending your hard-earned money on products that won't provide results. Plenty of snake oil salesmen will claim their creations will help grow your hair and nails, but if they actually had products that worked, wouldn't everybody know about them? Beauty is a big deal. If there were a hair-growth serum that worked, it would be the hottest item on the planet, and you probably wouldn't have any trouble finding it. The supplement biotin seems to go highly recommended for both hair and nail growth, but when I dug around for unbiased evidence that it actually worked, I couldn't find any. I've been taking it for years, and it has provided absolutely zero identifiable results. In fact, I think I'm going to stop wasting my money. Likely, the best thing you can do for your hair and nails is have patience … and a sense of humor. Time is truly the only real solution for this situation. And if you're willing to laugh at yourself, take some funny photos with your ever-changing appearance.

Brighten Your Days With …

Music. From pop to rock, country, rhythm, and blues, music has the power to make us FEEL. Feel happy, sad, emotional, excited, fearful, relaxed, and inspired. Use this tool from morning until night to boost your spirits, bring back fond memories, distract you from stress and add a little joy. Research has shown that music therapy can reduce stress and pain while increasing feelings of power.[20] Fill your playlists with these uplifting and inspiring songs to play when you're in the shower, car, cleaning, exercising, or in need of a boost of confidence and courage. These are some of my favorites.

- Tom Petty. "I Won't Back Down"
- Elton John. "I'm Still Standing"
- Rachel Platten. "Fight Song"
- Eminem. "Not Afraid"
- Kelly Clarkson. "Stronger"
- Travis Tritt. "It's a Great Day to Be Alive"
- Katrina and the Waves. "Walking On Sunshine"
- Rascal Flatts. "Stand"
- Journey. "Don't Stop Believing"
- Sia. "Unstoppable"
- Gloria Gaynor. "I Will Survive"
- Fleetwood Mac. "Don't Stop"

Art. In any form, art is commonly used to help people express their emotions. It's also a lot of fun and can be done in most stages of health and sickness. Whether you use a pencil, crayons, easel, clay, fabric, computer, or other mediums, getting creative is a clever way to boost your mood. And this works even if you consider yourself "unartistic" or "bad at art." Who cares what the final project looks like? Just enjoy the process. I highly suggest glitter be a part of all of your projects, but that's only because messes are fun too! You can complement your artful efforts by enjoying other people's art. Visiting art museums and galleries can serve as low-key entertainment in a temperature-controlled environment. You can also check out some phenomenal art galleries online.

Comedy. This may sound like a no-brainer, but intentionally pursuing laughter may make you … wait for it … happy! Alongside everything else you're doing to get well, laughter truly is the best medicine. Seek out comedy by spending time with your most hilarious friends, ditch dramatic movies and television shows for the funny stuff, listen to humorous podcasts, and find a local comedy club to enjoy live shows. I've said it before, you'll get zero extra points for being sad all the time. Make joy a priority!

Animals. Cute and cuddly, funny, awe-inspiring, and exciting, animals of all types can provide comfort, entertainment, and distractions. If you have pets, enjoy the comforts they bring. My dog never left my side when I was sick and her support made my situation much easier. If you don't have a pet and can get one, even a few fish can brighten your day. Take trips to the zoo or aquarium, visit friends with sweet pets, or ask your medical providers if they work with comfort animals. Animal-assisted therapy is a service offered at some cancer treatment facilities and hospitals. It can be extremely soothing to the patients. If you're stuck in a position where you cannot access animals in person, seek out funny animal videos on the internet. They're a wonderful distraction, and their complete innocence can be a real delight.

Friendship. Your pals are probably agonizing over your cancer diagnosis and wish they could help. LET THEM! Phone calls, video chats, and quality time together in person may be just what the doctor ordered. You do not have to do this alone, make time with others a priority. Isolation isn't good for anyone, so invite company over or get together for a meal, workout, or movie. If you truly do not know anyone in your area, join a local support group or join another type of club or class where you'll meet friends with similar interests. Engaging with others will go a long way to lift your spirits.

Sports. Whether you're playing or spectating, sports can add so much excitement, engagement, and purpose to your life. If you can play your favorite sport, keep doing so as much as possible. If you need to slow down from competition, but can still do something, do whatever you can. Play catch, drive balls at the range, serve tennis balls for someone else to gather, kick a soccer ball back and forth or play ping-pong. Even at a low level, sports are fun and do great things for your body. If you're not feeling up to participating, attend a live match, watch or listen to your favorite teams on the TV or radio, show up to watch some little league, or just watch biographies on your favorite teams and athletes. Sports are such a source of exhilaration and pride at any level, there should always be room for them in your life.

Go Outside! Nature is pretty magical. It's the only place fresh air can be found and exploring the great outdoors is a wonderful way to unplug from cancer, technology, politics, and drama. Connect with nature by venturing down a trail in the woods, or up a mountain. Spend time at the ocean, rivers, and lakes. Take a long drive through the desert with the windows down. You can even just sit on a blanket in your yard. That's right. A walk with your dog or time in a hammock can provide instant relief. Getting away from technology can be a powerful way to find peace within yourself. Whether you're feeling fantastic or sluggish, get outside multiple times each day.

Read. Escape inside the pages of mysteries, romance novels, adventure, self-help books, and more. A good book can carry you through all sorts of adventures, serving to entertain, distract, educate and enlighten. Flip or swipe through the pages on your couch or in the many waiting rooms you visit. Make your selection experience part of the fun; perusing bookstores and libraries can be really enjoyable.

Strawberry Moments. Acknowledge the sweetest parts of each day by discussing them with your loved ones or writing them down in your *Healthy Cancer Comeback Journal*. Focusing on the silver linings in this weird world of cancer can lift your spirits and help you maintain perspective. Cancer completely sucks, but there are still incredible experiences to enjoy. Don't just think about them, choose at least three and bask in them by talking with anyone who will listen or jot them down. The longer your list of strawberry moments, the better!

Spa & Beauty Day. Whether you do it at home or in a salon, pampering yourself with treatments like facials, manicures, pedicures, and massages can work wonders. It feels fabulous when a professional provides these services, but it can also feel fab when you do them yourself or with some friends. You may also want to spend some time trying out new hair and makeup skills if your appearance has changed since your treatment began. I leaned on instructional YouTube videos for guidance when I lost my eyebrows and eyelashes, which were very helpful! My major find was "eyebrow stamps," look them up if you need them. If you wear wigs, perhaps you can try some new colors and styles to mix things up. Dedicate time to self-care without feeling guilty. You deserve this!

Retail Therapy. Even on a budget, shopping can be an awesome way to boost your mood and a great way to stay active. Whether you're looking for a stylish outfit or cool end tables, shopping can be very cathartic. If you can't make it to a store physically, look online. If shopping online, you'll get to enjoy the excitement twice: at the time of purchase and when it arrives.

Creative Cooking. If your tummy feels strange or your taste buds are on strike, try out a few new recipes. Many people cook and bake for fun, so this might be a multi-purpose victory. A. You may find something that your stomach tolerates and your mouth enjoys. B. You may delight in the experience of cutting, stirring, blending, etc … C. You fill your tummy with food.

Brain Training. Chemo Brain is real. I speak from experience on the subject. Chemotherapy, surgeries, radiation, and pharmaceuticals can leave patients confused, forgetful, or lacking the ability to concentrate. The medical community has dubbed it "cancer-induced cognitive impairment" and up to 70-percent of cancer patients report some level of deterioration in cognitive function following chemotherapy. Sure your brain is an organ, but if you train it like a muscle it may respond similarly. A University of Sydney study has shown that "brain training" games targeting attention, memory, and visual skills reduced chemotherapy-induced neurological problems in cancer patients.[21] Build brain training into your days with crossword puzzles, word games, brainteasers, and math. Whether you utilize paper or digital games, there is no downside to spending 10 minutes a day doing so and some of these challenges are pretty fun.

Learn Something New. The thrill of trying and conquering unchartered territories feels pretty great, and when it comes to productive learning, any option will do. Learn a new dance move, a few words in a foreign language, or how to fix something. The idea is to constantly be working on becoming more than you are. Even if it feels like cancer is dragging you down, you can always do something to lift yourself up. Learning something new doesn't have to mean reaching a new major goal— it can simply mean reading an interesting fact or immersing yourself in a fascinating subject.

Go for a Long Drive. Getting in the car and getting "out" might be the perfect option for days when you don't feel like being active. Find a scenic route or just roll down the windows and bask in the feeling of wind on your face.

Game Night. Being at home doesn't have to be boring, especially with a few of your favorite people, a deck of cards, puzzles, or board games. Set things up on the kitchen table or around the couch and laugh your heads off.

Arcade. Pinball, ski ball, and air hockey are staples at every arcade. These plus other games make an arcade a creative choice for being in temperature controlled environment, with both active and stationary activities. Even though online gamers make "games" sound complicated, the arcade variety is still pretty easy to enjoy without much skill. Consider the opportunity to earn tickets to exchange for unimpressive prizes or candy as a bonus.

CHAPTER ELEVEN

Your cancer crushing community

Stealing independence is one of the rudest maneuvers cancer makes. For many of us, asking for or accepting help can be just as challenging as sitting down for chemo. It certainly made me very uncomfortable. Even though I'd supported many friends battling cancer in the past, when it was my turn, I cringed. "I'm a helper, not a helpee," I thought. However, when things went sideways and sickness prevented me from driving safely, shopping, cooking, and cleaning, I had to reevaluate. Besides my own needs, my children needed rides to school and activities, meals, and more. I was fortunate to have a caring husband, but he had a full-time job. As awkward as it was to accept support, I chose to welcome it graciously with a commitment to spending the rest of my life paying it forward to help others.

A stubborn streak is going to benefit your cancer battle in a million ways. Refusing to give up, staying committed to fitness, and pursuing things that make you happy are signs of strength. Refusing to allow friends to drop off meals or groceries won't make you strong though, it will make you foolish. Rejecting an offer from a neighbor who'd like to mow your lawn after your surgery is just dumb. If you can't accept support and feel good about it, choose to accept support knowing the person helping you will feel good about it. As you know, watching someone you care about fight cancer can make you feel powerless. When friends get to pitch in and do something to make a cancer patient's life easier, it makes them feel powerful. If you can't accept help graciously for your own benefit, do it for theirs.

When people tell you to let them know if you need help, they mean it. There are also local nonprofits all over the world dedicated to providing support for cancer patients. Like your friends, they can provide all sorts of helpful resources and I implore you not to be too prideful to ask. We know that cancer can cause suffering. Don't let your ego make a bad situation worse. Be compassionate with yourself and utilize all resources when necessary.

Note to Caregivers

Yes, I'm talking to YOU! If you're reading this hoping to help your favorite Cancer Crushing Friend (CCF) … thank you. You're clearly a smart, generous, and caring soul. I appreciate you. Your role can be tremendously important to your CCF's success, both short-term and long-term. There's a laundry list of ways you can help, which will vary depending on whether you live in the same home or town, or live on opposite ends of the earth. To review some ideas, let's break help down into a few categories.

Functional. This type of help encompasses your CCF's basic needs. Food, water, shelter, transportation, and medicine. Some CCFs have this stuff covered with no problem, but many do not. Offer rides to appointments, meals, shopping, dog-walking, housecleaning, and yard mowing. Driving isn't ideal for a patient under the influence of medications, and I've heard stories of people missing appointments for treatments because they couldn't catch a ride or afford gas. Terrible. So look around and see what needs to be done. Do the manual labor yourself, bring extra friends into the mix when necessary, or hire someone to help if you can. Hiring professionals to do house cleaning, food delivery, yard work, and transportation is a fantastic way for out-of-towners to provide support.

Since we're excited about your CCF's healthy cancer comeback, it would be fabulous to offer support in fitness. Get together to walk, dance, stretch, swim, or strength train. Meet at the gym, take a class or go canoeing. Having a partner will inspire your CCF to show up, work a little harder and enjoy the process even more. You may also be the type of partner who makes sure your CCF doesn't work too hard, stays hydrated, doesn't fall down, and serves as a safety net. Depending on where they are in their treatment and recovery will determine what role you need to play.

Financial. Medical expenses can add up, and loss of work can be devastating. Gift cards are a thoughtful way to offer financial support without the recipient feeling like they are receiving a handout. Gift cards are GIFTS! Receiving one feels totally different than receiving cash. Gift cards for groceries, gas, food delivery services, online shopping, or rides can be used for essentials. You can also send gift cards for movies, restaurants, fitness classes, spas, or streaming services to inspire quality time outside of the home or entertainment when your CCF is stuck in bed. A generic Visa or American Express gift card can be used wherever credit cards are accepted, and when put inside a cute get-well-soon card, is far easier to receive than cash. Lastly, if your CCF is facing a catastrophic financial crisis, setting up a crowdfunding page online with their permission could be very helpful.

Emotional. The stress that comes along with cancer is unlike any other. Even if it appears your CCF is handling treatment with ease, I assure you, there are likely tears and anxiety behind the scenes. You can alleviate this by escorting your CCF to appointments. While providing comfort and companionship, an extra pair of ears can provide clarity on what was discussed during appointments. Take lots of notes, because it's all very easy to forget or confuse. Committing to being a consistent and caring presence in your CCF's life can go a long way. Talking about cancer can be comforting and talking about everything besides cancer can be a wonderful distraction. Hopefully, you'll know how and when to mix things up.

Without becoming overbearing, stop by for social visits, call regularly, and include your CCF in fun social activities as often as possible. Make outings easier by stopping by to pick your CCF up. Far-away friends can send regular cards, emails, and texts. A few special friends of mine would often text "Please don't feel obligated to reply, just know that I love you." Receiving permission not to respond removed a lot of pressure on the days when I was super sick. Even if you're not a traditionally sunny person, show up with a smile on your face and find ways to make your CCF's day brighter. While it's definitely okay to cry together, basking in grief can be counterproductive. Your friendship can comfort, support, entertain, and distract.

This is a strange concept to have to suggest, but do not ghost your CCF! Cancer Ghosting is a bizarre phenomenon that happened to me and apparently happens to many other people. When I was diagnosed, people came out of the woodwork to offer support and kindness, which was very appreciated. Strangely, a couple of my lifelong BFFs completely disappeared without sending so much as a text to tell me they cared. It was sad, to say the least. Since you're reading this, you likely aren't the type of person to disappear on a CCF, which I appreciate. Just know that even if you're scared for your CCF or feel like you're in the way, your love will always be appreciated.

Cancer is not something a person should have to fight alone. Thank you for using your cancer-crushing abilities to empower your Cancer Crushing Friend!

Gifts of Service
- Rides
- Pick up prescriptions
- Organize meal delivery from friends/neighbors
- Buy groceries
- Housecleaning
- Laundry

- Ironing
- Errands
- Shopping
- Dog-walking
- Pet care
- Car cleaning
- Auto maintenance
- Help manage bills
- Spend time together
- Go to appointments together
- Take notes at appointments
- Wash hair
- Clip nails
- Be an exercise buddy
- Lawn maintenance

Gifts Cards and Gifts of Monetary Value

- Groceries
- Gas
- Rideshare Services/Taxi
- Restaurants
- Movies
- Shows
- Streaming services
- Spa services
- House cleaning services
- Gym Membership
- Movie theater passes
- Adventure pass
- Museum pass
- American Express/Visa Gift Card
- Online shopping
- Audiobook subscription

- Music streaming subscription
- Crowdfunding

Tangible Gifts

- Gift basket filled with lots of goodies.
- Cozy blankets
- Neck pillow
- Soft bedding
- Hats/caps/beanies
- Scarves
- Healthy snacks
- Board games
- Puzzles
- Books
- Madlibs
- Hypoallergenic moisturizing lotions
- Hypoallergenic lip-balms
- Massage tools
- Heating pads
- Soft ice packs
- Medical devices like shower chairs if needed
- Water bottles
- Thank you notes and a pretty pen
- Craft supplies
- *Healthy Cancer Comeback Journal*

YOU CAN DO **HARD THINGS**

Friend, I am incredibly proud of you. When cancer showed up, bringing overwhelming feelings of fear and helplessness, you sought to fight back with knowledge and power. You chose to be a victor instead of a victim, and that makes you a total badass. The control you have over your own well-being is undeniable. Paired with care from scientists and medical providers, your personal efforts toward health are going to make this experience both easier and less horrible. As I suffered and soared during my 15 months of treatment for breast cancer, my oncologist repeatedly reminded me that I was only able to travel, work and play because of my commitment to health. He also stressed that my suffering would have been far worse without it. That stuck with me, and I hope it sticks with you.

You can do hard things! Make the voice in your head an enthusiastic coach and cheerleader who believes in you above all else and remind yourself that you are fierce every single day. Do so when you set out to exercise, and especially when cancer tries to intimidate you. This, paired with a commitment to perspective, passions, and positivity will be the strength your brain needs to keep your body moving in the right direction. It's not so complicated. You have to believe in YOU!

Set ambitious goals for yourself physically, and do your best to stick with thoughtful strategies to reach them. If you need to detour because times get tough, show compassion for yourself and move forward with alternate plans. Remember, doing something is better than doing nothing. Choose foods that help instead of hurt more often than not, and make that bottle of water your constant companion. Perfection is impossible to achieve with nutrition, but aim to make mostly great choices. You'll be surprised by the benefits you reap when you feed your body foods designed to make it thrive.

When the hardest part of cancer care is over, I hope you choose to live larger than ever before. With a radical new understanding that life truly is short, make the most of each day by doing things that make you feel the most alive. Travel, adventure, challenge yourself athletically, seek out new experiences, advance your career or retire, forgive, love, sing karaoke, and dance in the freaking rain! Conquering cancer makes many of us fearless, which is absolutely freeing. Think about it, after facing the big "C," what's so scary about the mundane challenges one might face in the real world? I assure you, moving forward, everything else in your life will feel strikingly easier. Whether it be in sports, social situations, work, or leisure, you may find yourself living braver and bolder than you did previously.

Most importantly, I hope you commit to doing better and being better. Make your future a lifetime celebration of Your Healthy Cancer Comeback!

I'M ROOTING FOR YOU!

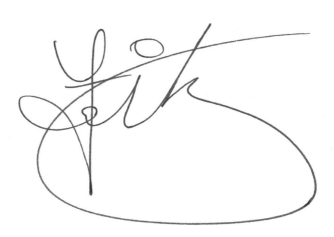

Acknowledgments

My cancer-crushing friends. Even though we're part of a club we never wanted to be in, it sure is cool to have each other for inspiration, information, and support. Fight hard, commit to health, immerse yourself in things that bring you joy, and be persistent. I believe in you!

Big love to my family, who has tolerated my many hours on my laptop. You're each always striving for greatness, and it's pretty exciting to be a part of that.

Huge smooches and snuggles to my doggos, Piper and Joey, who provide me with endless joy, laughter, and comfort. Piper is the ultimate best friend and never left my side when I was sick. She has also shined as vice president of my company Fitzness International. I will spend the rest of her days making her feel happy, comfortable, and loved. Joey has added so much sweet and silly joy to my life, and the two always give me the perfect incentive to step away from my laptop and go outside for some fresh air and fun. On behalf of all the Pipers and Joeys who need a home, readers, please rescue them!

Rudy Novotny, thank you for always going above and beyond to support, guide, and cheer for me. You are so much more than just the most talented, big-voiced announcer in endurance sports. Your contributions to my books have been immeasurable. #TeamNoisy

Dr. Dawn Mussallem and Dr. Allison Grow. Thank you both for taking time out of your incredibly busy and important days caring for cancer patients to read and provide feedback and support for this book. I adore and admire you both.

Tara Gidus Collingwood, MS, RDN. Thanks for sharing your nutrition expertise and up-close-and-personal experience as a caregiver for your late husband. You're a total pro, and I'm grateful to have you as a friend and colleague.

My Beta Readers. Thanks for reading this book in advance to share your thoughts and suggestions, to help me make it great. I hate that most of us have endured cancer, but I'm grateful this nasty disease has brought us together. Your contributions enable me to help the next generation of patients and survivors to live better and longer. Phil Decker, Kathie Bieritz, Kelly Ryan, Tamara Milliken, Michael Jones, Victoria Mikko, Chris Voss, and Rudy Novotny.

My personal oncology team: Dr. Lucio Gordan, Dr. Cherryle Hayes, and Dr. Peter Sarantos. It's never a bad time to thank you for saving my life. You each provided world-class care and never tried to stop me from living fully during my treatment. I love you.

My Noisy Cancer Comeback readers. Thanks for the constant positive feedback and for committing to improving your life with perspective, passion, and positivity. It thrills me to see you living joyfully and enthusiastically conquering hard things.

My Fitzness fiends and Hotties. Helping you live better and longer excites me to no end. Thanks for trusting me and for doing the things that make you better. You are worth my effort and your own!

My running community. You fill me with constant joy and brightened my days when cancer tried to make them dark. I'll be forever grateful for us and promise to continue making happy noise and exchanging sweaty hugs at your start and finish lines. I love you.

Paige Douglass. Thank you for sharing your time and expertise as a cancer rehabilitation specialist. I'm in awe of your extraordinary athleticism as a cancer patient. You are proof that fitness is possible! #BostonBuddies

Mom. Thanks for raising me right, loving me lots, and always cheering me on. Our daily FaceTime chats make me happy. I love you.

John. Your entrepreneurial spirit is incredible, and that's just one of many reasons you're my favorite brother. #TheFitz #TheFitzness

Kristi Hill. You make me happy, FunPig.

Alicia Wilcox. I appreciate your talent.

Rob Middaugh. My physical therapist. Thanks for using your big brain and evil thumbs to help me make my healthy cancer comeback.

Alex Muknicka. Your incredible massages and stretches were a huge force in helping me get back to being athletic. Thank you.

Doug Thurston. Your proofreading is second only to your race directing and third only to your whale calls.

Jennifer Jeffres Sen. I appreciate you turning your big brain on to proofread my book. I love you and your pretty toenails.

Melissa Redon. My graphic designer and friend. I knew you'd create the bold, vibrant, happy book designs I craved. Thank you!

Phil Stokes. Thanks for introducing yourself to me at the gym years ago and offering to take some professional photos for me. Besides being a wildly talented photographer, you are such a decent man.

My Fitzness Interns. Omar Benitez, Jeremy Taylor, Devin Thompson, Garrett Gerard, and Jill Quigley. Thank you for being a part of my team. I'm so grateful for your talents, efforts, ingenuity, and contributions to the success of this book. Go Gators!

To my American Military, Veterans and First Responders. I'll never miss an opportunity to thank you for your service, sacrifice, and protection of our freedoms. I am forever grateful.

Citations

1. Sheinboim, Danna, Shivang Parikh, Paulee Manich, Irit Markus, Sapir Dahan, Roma Parikh, Elisa Stubbs, et al. "An Exercise-Induced Metabolic Shield in Distant Organs Blocks Cancer Progression and Metastatic Dissemination." Cancer Research 82, no. 22 (2022): 4164–78. https://doi.org/10.1158/0008-5472.can-22-0237.

2. McTiernan, Anne, Christine M Friedenreich, Peter T Katzmarzyk, Kenneth E Powell, Richard Macko, David Buchner, Linda S Pescatello, et al. "Physical Activity in Cancer Prevention and Survival: A Systematic Review." Medicine and science in sports and exercise. U.S. National Library of Medicine, June 2019. https://www.ncbi.nlm.nih.gov/pmc/articles/PMC6527123/.PAGE6

3. Koehler, Fitz, and Dawn Mussallem. Effects of exercise and quality nutrition on cancer. Personal, April 18, 2022.

4. Moreland, Briana, Ramakrishna Kakara, and Ankita Henry. "Trends in Nonfatal Falls and Fall-Related Injuries among Adults Aged ≥65 Years — United States, 2012–2018." MMWR. Morbidity and Mortality Weekly Report 69, no. 27 (2020): 875–81. https://doi.org/10.15585/mmwr.mm6927a5.

5. "Eat a Diet Rich in Whole Grains, Vegetables, Fruits, and Beans." American Institute for Cancer Research, January 26, 2021. https://www.aicr.org/cancer-prevention/recommendations/eat-a-diet-rich-in-whole-grains-vegetables-fruits-and-beans/#what-the-science-says.

6. "Cancer: Carcinogenicity of the Consumption of Red Meat and Processed Meat." World Health Organization. World Health Organization, October 26, 2015. https://www.aicr.org/cancer-prevention/food-facts/red-meat-beef-pork-lamb/.

7. World Health Organization. "Cancer: Carcinogenicity of the Consumption of Red Meat and Processed Meat." Accessed January 1, 2023. https://www.who.int/news-room/questions-and-answers/item/cancer-carcinogenicity-of-the-consumption-of-red-meat-and-processed-meat

8. Center for Food Safety and Applied Nutrition. "Final Determination Regarding Partially Hydrogenated Oils." U.S. Food and Drug Administration. FDA, May 18, 2018. https://www.fda.gov/food/food-additives-petitions/final-determination-regarding-partially-hydrogenated-oils-removing-trans-fat.

9. American Heart Association Editorial Staff. "Saturated Fat." www.heart.org, July 20, 2022. https://www.heart.org/en/healthy-living/healthy-eating/eat-smart/fats/saturated-fats.

10. U.S. Department of Health and Human Services and U.S. Department of Agriculture. "Dietary Guidelines for Americans 2015-2020 8th Edition ." 2015–2020 Dietary Guidelines for Americans. 8th Edition. . The U.S. Department of Health and Human Services , December 1, 2015. https://health.gov/our-work/nutrition-physical-activity/dietary-guidelines/previous-dietary-guidelines/2015. 3.

11. "Eat a Diet Rich in Whole Grains, Vegetables, Fruits, and Beans." American Institute for Cancer Research, January 26, 2021. https://www.aicr.org/cancer-prevention/recommendations/eat-a-diet-rich-in-whole-grains-vegetables-fruits-and-beans/#what-the-science-says.

12. "Pulses: Dry Beans, Peas, and Lentils (Legumes)." American Institute for Cancer Research. American Institute for Cancer Research , August 3,

2021. https://www.aicr.org/cancer-prevention/food-facts/dry-beans-and-peas-legumes/.13. Polak, Rani, Edward M. Phillips, and Amy Campbell. "Legumes: Health Benefits and Culinary Approaches to Increase Intake." Clinical Diabetes 33, no. 4 (2015): 198–205. https://doi.org/10.2337/diaclin.33.4.198.

14. Mitchell, H. H., T. S. Hamilton, F. R. Steggerda, and H. W. Bean. "The Chemical Composition of the Adult Human Body and Its Bearing on the Biochemistry of Growth." Journal of Biological Chemistry 158, no. 3 (1945): 625-637. https://doi.org/10.1016/S0021-9258(19)51339-4.

15. Fiolet, Thibault, Bernard Srour, Laury Sellem, Emmanuelle Kesse-Guyot, Benjamin Allès, Caroline Méjean, Mélanie Deschasaux, et al. "Consumption of Ultra-Processed Foods and Cancer Risk: Results from NutriNet-Santé Prospective Cohort." BMJ 360, no. 322 (February 14, 2018). https://doi.org/10.1136/bmj.k322.

16. "Alcohol and Cancer." Division of Cancer Prevention and Control, Centers for Disease Control and Prevention, January 31, 2022. https://www.cdc.gov/cancer/alcohol/index.htm.

17. "Does Sugar Feed Cancer?" Dana-Farber Cancer Institute, 2023. https://www.dana-farber.org/for-patients-and-families/care-and-treatment/support-services-and-amenities/nutrition-services/faqs/sugar-and-cancer/.

18. Koehler, Fitz, and Allison Grow. Interview with Dr. Allison Grow, MD, PhD. Other, n.d.

19. Koehler, Fitz, and Dawn Mussallem. Effects of exercise and quality nutrition on cancer. Personal, April 18, 2022.

20. Thoma, Myriam V., Roberto La Marca, Rebecca Brönnimann, Linda Finkel, Ulrike Ehlert, and Urs M. Nater. "The Effect of Music on the Human Stress Response." PLoS ONE 8, no. 8 (2013). https://doi.org/10.1371/journal.pone.0070156.

21. Bray, Victoria J., Haryana M. Dhillon, Melanie L. Bell, Michael Kabourakis, Mallorie H. Fiero, Desmond Yip, Frances Boyle, Melanie A. Price, and Janette L. Vardy. "Evaluation of a Web-Based Cognitive Rehabilitation Program in Cancer Survivors Reporting Cognitive Symptoms after Chemotherapy." Journal of Clinical Oncology 35, no. 2 (2017): 217–25. https://doi.org/10.1200/jco.2016.67.8201.

Advanced Praise

"*Your Health Cancer Comeback: Sick to Strong* is chock full of information and inspiration. Fitz's knowledge, enthusiasm, and desire for everyone to gain or regain control of their health comes through loud and clear. This book is exactly what you need to come back stronger and healthier than ever."

—**Kathleen Bieritz, Stage 2 Breast Cancer Survivor**

"*Your Healthy Cancer Comeback: Sick to Strong* is a comprehensive how-to guide that addresses the critical importance of a healthy lifestyle during and after a cancer diagnosis. Fitz breaks down complex evidence-based scientific facts into a patient-centered, easy-to-understand guide filled with actionable pearls on how to live your best life during and after a cancer diagnosis. This empowering go-to source will, without a doubt, motivate you to live a healthy life, move you from "sick to strong," and help to improve cancer outcomes!"

—**Dawn Mussallem, DO, DipABLM**
  Lifestyle Medicine Breast Physician

"This is a brilliant tutorial on how to take your health and life back during and after overcoming cancer. Fitz breaks it down and makes living a healthy life simple with tips on exercise, nutrition, hydration, sleep, and more! If you want to learn to thrive and not just survive, read this book!"

—**Tara Collingwood, MS, RDN, CSSD, LD/N, ACSM-CPT**
  Board Certified Sports Dietitian

"Whether you're being treated for cancer, have been treated for cancer—or simply hope never to NEED cancer treatment—*Your Healthy Cancer Comeback: Sick to Strong* is your inspiration and practical guide. Life brings us all kinds of unanticipated difficulties, with cancer at the scarier end of that list. When you don't know how you're going to get through it, Fitz Koehler is here to remind you that "you can do hard things" and to break it down for you. No matter how hard cancer knocks you down, she shows you how to make a start, how to keep it going, and how to end up better than before. I love her approach because it's eminently practical and straightforward and because she's a survivor and thriver. Wherever you are, she's been there and climbed out. I also love it because it's for everyone--you don't have to be young, commit to a specific kind of diet, or aspire to be an elite athlete. You just have to want to live and live well. It's also fun and easy to read. What are you waiting for? Buy it now!"

—Dr. Allison Grow, MD, PhD
   Radiation Oncologist

"Mindset and determination are important keys to achieving your best outcomes after a cancer diagnosis. *Your Healthy Cancer Comeback: Sick to Strong* provides a precise roadmap for patients and caregivers during a difficult time. Fitz Koehler's work is filled with experience and explanation to assist all throughout the journey. Fully recommend!"

—David Kashmer, MD MBA FACS
   Surgeon

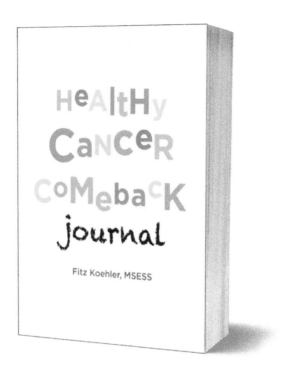

Cancer is complicated, emotional, challenging, and filled with unique moments. Filled with thoughtful prompts, keep track of your experiences in oncology, along with your feelings, fears, laughter, tears, faith, and facts about your care. Document your strategies for exercise, nutrition, and progress on your way from sick to strong.

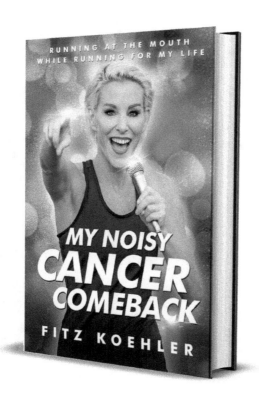

"A funny, dramatic, and honest insight into one very noisy woman's adventures and misadventures while battling cancer. It's the ultimate motivational tool for thriving while surviving! Fitz's story proves that anyone can endure hardships better by utilizing perspective, passion, and positivity."

Cancer Comeback 3-pack

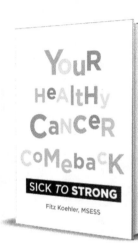
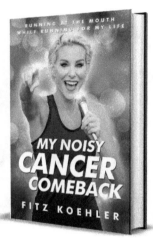
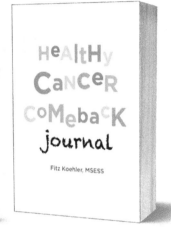

The Cancer Comeback Series is packed with inspiration and information every cancer patient and survivor needs to go from sick to strong! Makes a great gift.

Signed copies and bulk orders available at Fitzness.com

FiTzNeSS.COM

The Fitzness Show
Recipes
Workout Videos
Articles
Training Tips
Fitz's Event Calendar
Books and Online Courses
Cancer Comeback Stories- submit yours!
Inspirational Cancer Comeback Gear
Contact Fitz

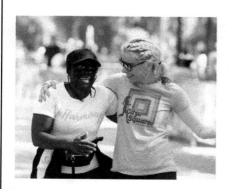

FiTzNeSS.COM

Home   Meet Fitz | Race Announcer | Keynote Speaker | Fitzness Blog | TV/Podcast Appearances | Workout Videos | The Fitzness Show | Fitz vs. Breast Cancer | Morning Mile

LIVE BETTER AND LONGER

Motivational Keynote Presentations

Energetic. Entertaining. Compelling.

Book Fitz at Fitzness.com

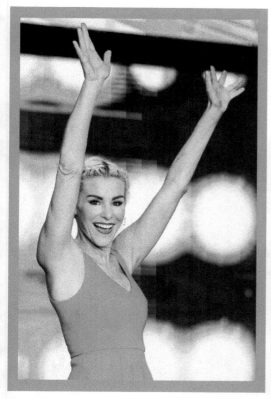

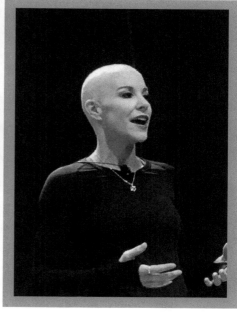

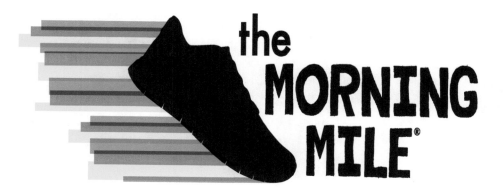

The Morning Mile™ is an easily-implemented before-school walking/running program that gives children a chance to start each day in an active way while enjoying fun, music, and friends. That's EVERY CHILD, EVERY DAY. It's also supported by a wonderful system of rewards, which keeps students highly motivated and frequently congratulated. Inquire to sponsor programs or to get your favorite schools started.

Let's Get More Kids Moving in The Mornings!

MORNINGMILE.COM

Let's Connect!

FITZNESS on Facebook
@Fitzness on Instagram
@Fitzness on YouTube
Fitz Koehler on Linkedin
Fitzness13 on TikTok
HealthyCancerComeback on Instragram

#FITZNESS
#HealthyCancerComeback

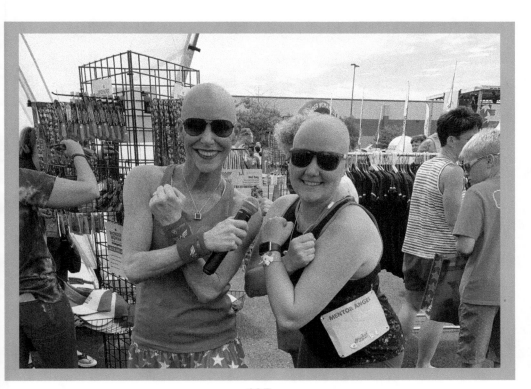

About the Author

Fitz Koehler is among the most prominent and compelling fitness experts and race announcers in America. With a Master's Degree in Exercise and Sport Sciences and decades of experience teaching fitness worldwide, Fitz has helped countless people live better and longer by making fitness understandable, attainable, and fun. As CEO of Fitzness International, she masterfully uses every form of mass media to lead people toward health and athletic adventure.

In 2019, Fitz was diagnosed with breast cancer, and her healthy and athletic body was brutalized by 15 months of chemotherapy, radiation, and surgeries. Instead of shutting down, she turned the volume up on her career. She also strategically orchestrated her own healthy cancer comeback from sick, scrawny, and weak to a strong Boston Marathon finisher. Her memoir *My Noisy Cancer Comeback: Running at the Mouth, While Running for My Life* was released in 2020 and has been a massive source of motivation for those facing hardships of all sorts. Fitz shares inspirational lessons from her cancer-crushing whirlwind in her keynote presentations, convincing global audiences that they "can do hard things," too.

As the voice of the Los Angeles Marathon, Buffalo Marathon, Big Sur Marathon, Detroit Free Press Marathon, DC Super Hero Series, and more, Fitz brings big structure, energy, and joy to sports. She has appeared on many national media outlets, hosts a popular podcast, The Fitzness Show, and has performed as a speaker and spokesperson for corporations like Disney®, Oakley®, Tropicana®, and Office Depot®. Fitz's successful school running/walking program, The Morning Mile®, has inspired millions of children, their families, and teachers to get moving in the mornings.

In her free time, Fitz enjoys water sports, strength training, obstacle course races, animals, hugs, sarcasm, getting muddy in her Jeep Wrangler, and travel. She lives in Gainesville, Florida.

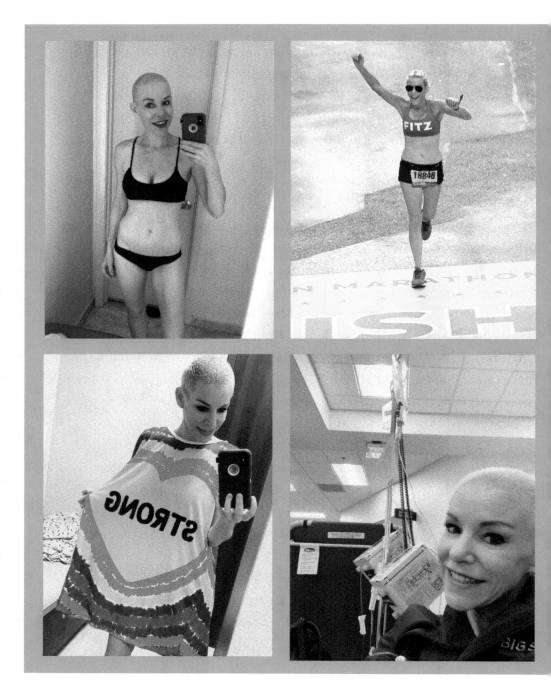

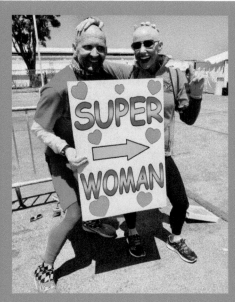

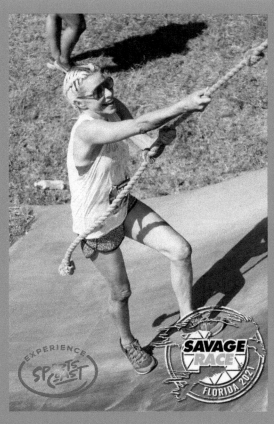

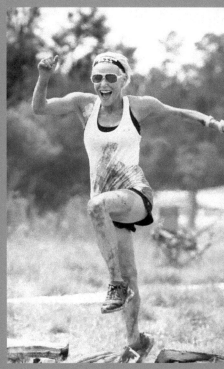

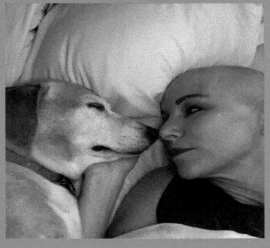

Printed in the USA
CPSIA information can be obtained
at www.ICGtesting.com
LVHW020636250124
R18036700001B/R180367PG769489LVX00002B/1